MW00439473

Just Enough Physiology

MAYO CLINIC SCIENTIFIC PRESS

Mayo Clinic Atlas of Regional Anesthesia and Ultrasound-Guided Nerve Blockade
Edited by James R. Hebl, MD, and Robert L. Lennon, DO

Mayo Clinic Preventive Medicine and Public Health Board Review
Edited by Prathibha Varkey, MBBS, MPH, MHPE

Mayo Clinic Internal Medicine Board Review, Ninth Edition
Edited by Amit K. Ghosh, MD

Mayo Clinic Challenging Images for Pulmonary Board Review
Edward C. Rosenow III, MD

Mayo Clinic Gastroenterology and Hepatology Board Review, Fourth Edition
Edited by Stephen C. Hauser, MD

Mayo Clinic Infectious Diseases Board Review
Edited by Zelalem Temesgen, MD

Mayo Clinic Antimicrobial Handbook: Quick Guide, Second Edition
Edited by John W. Wilson, MD, and Lynn L. Estes, PharmD

Just Enough Physiology

JAMES R. MUNIS, MD, PhD
Consultant
Division of Neuroanesthesia
and Department of Physiology
and Biomedical Engineering
Mayo Clinic;
Assistant Professor of
Anesthesiology and of Physiology
College of Medicine
Mayo Clinic
Rochester, Minnesota

MAYO CLINIC SCIENTIFIC PRESS   OXFORD UNIVERSITY PRESS

MAYO
CLINIC

The triple-shield Mayo logo and the words MAYO, MAYO CLINIC, and MAYO CLINIC SCIENTIFIC PRESS
are marks of Mayo Foundation for Medical Education and Research.

OXFORD
UNIVERSITY PRESS

Oxford University Press, Inc., publishes works that further
Oxford University's objective of excellence
in research, scholarship, and education.

Oxford   New York
Auckland   Cape Town   Dar es Salaam   Hong Kong   Karachi
Kuala Lumpur   Madrid   Melbourne   Mexico City   Nairobi
New Delhi   Shanghai   Taipei   Toronto

With offices in
Argentina   Austria   Brazil   Chile   Czech Republic   France   Greece
Guatemala   Hungary   Italy   Japan   Poland   Portugal   Singapore
South Korea   Switzerland   Thailand   Turkey   Ukraine   Vietnam

Copyright © 2012 by Mayo Foundation for Medical Education and Research.

Published by Oxford University Press, Inc.
198 Madison Avenue, New York, New York 10016
www.oup.com

Oxford is a registered trademark of Oxford University Press

All rights reserved. No part of this publication may be reproduced, stored in a retrieval system, or transmitted,
in any form or by any means, electronic, mechanical, photocopying, recording, or otherwise, without
the prior permission of Mayo Foundation for Medical Education and Research. Inquiries should be addressed
to Scientific Publications, Plummer 10, Mayo Clinic, 200 First St SW, Rochester, MN 55905

Library of Congress Cataloging-in-Publication Data
Munis, James R.
Just enough physiology / James R. Munis.
p. ; cm.
ISBN 978–0–19–979779–0 (pbk.)
I. Title.
[DNLM: 1. Physiological Phenomena. QT 4]
LC classification not assigned
612.1—dc23   2011030222

Mayo Foundation does not endorse any particular products or services, and the reference to any products or services
in this book is for informational purposes only and should not be taken as an endorsement by the authors or Mayo
Foundation. Care has been taken to confirm the accuracy of the information presented and to describe generally accepted
practices. However, the authors, editors, and publisher are not responsible for errors or omissions or for any consequences
from application of the information in this book and make no warranty, express or implied, with respect to the contents of
the publication. This book should not be relied on apart from the advice of a qualified health care provider.

The authors, editors, and publisher have exerted efforts to ensure that drug selection and dosage set forth in this text are
in accordance with current recommendations and practice at the time of publication. However, in view of ongoing research,
changes in government regulations, and the constant flow of information relating to drug therapy and drug reactions, readers
are urged to check the package insert for each drug for any change in indications and dosage and for added wordings and
precautions. This is particularly important when the recommended agent is a new or infrequently employed drug.

Some drugs and medical devices presented in this publication have US Food and Drug Administration (FDA)
clearance for limited use in restricted research settings. It is the responsibility of the health care providers
to ascertain the FDA status of each drug or device planned for use in their clinical practice.

9 8 7 6 5 4 3 2 1

Printed in China
on acid-free paper

For Lisa

PREFACE

THIS BOOK EMERGED FROM a long tradition of one-on-one teaching, and I hope it reads that way. What began as notes on chalkboards and scraps of paper eventually became a teaching monograph. These essays, aided and abetted by various illustrations and observations, were used as a core resource for a second-year physiology course at Mayo Medical School, starting in 2002. It was also used since that time as a handout for rotating and visiting residents in anesthesiology and critical care. Following a kind and enthusiastic recognition by the Anesthesia Foundation in 2008, Oxford University Press and Mayo Clinic Scientific Press have shaped *Just Enough Physiology* into a real textbook. My own illustrations have been replaced with the far more professional work of James Tidwell, and each essay has been edited and rewritten, but with an emphasis on preserving a consistent voice. I say "essay" because that is really what each chapter is—a story. People remember stories longer than they do arguments, equations, or concepts. So, by embedding arguments, equations, and concepts—the necessary stuff of physiology—within stories, I hope that you will learn more and remember more.

For more than 2 decades, I have taught what I hope have been a few surprising but useful concepts about cardiopulmonary physiology to college, medical, and other professional students in the classroom, as well as to residents and fellows in the operating room and hospital. Like many other teachers, I have discovered that our brains can hold only so much at one time. That is why *Just Enough Physiology* is divided into small, easily digested topics. I have kept each one short in the hope that you will be able to dine on an entire topic at one sitting and still have room for dessert. Left to our own devices as teachers and students, I believe that is how we best learn, remember, and apply.

In one sense, *Just Enough Physiology* takes an inverted approach to teaching. Many textbooks are written explicitly for board preparation and hope to sneak in some real science along the way. This book will do just the opposite: it will take you by the hand through some of the theory, history, and quirky places where the science of physiology makes its home (Mt Everest, Mars, or beneath the sea, for example); preparing you to answer questions is an imperceptible side benefit. By way of reassurance (but without making any extraordinary claim to comprehensiveness), I think you are unlikely to field questions about the physiology of the heart, lungs, or circulation that *Just Enough Physiology* doesn't equip you to answer. Most of what you need to know for the boards or on rounds is in here somewhere.

One of my mentors during my postgraduate training was Dr Richard Teplick at the Massachusetts General Hospital. He taught a year-long physiology and pathophysiology course for critical care fellows that began with Newton's Laws of Motion. Dr Lawrence Wood did the same at the University of Chicago. The benefit of beginning at the beginning—that is, with basic physical principles—cannot be overstated. Physiology is the science that is applied at the boundary between life and death; this is why it's so important to those of us who tread that same boundary every day in the practice of anesthesiology and critical care. The functional difference between a patient who has just died and one who is still alive is physiology.

What the heart, lungs, and circulation do in life is best understood through some simple, unifying principles of mechanics and chemistry. But that is not enough. There is also a way of thinking about these concepts that helps pull them together. Interestingly, that form of logic is almost identical to the way our brains work when we are solving logic puzzles. To that effect, brain teasers are included at the end of each chapter. I hope that your brain is both enriched and teased as you work your way through these stories.

James Munis, MD, PhD
Rochester, Minnesota

ACKNOWLEDGMENTS

I HAVE BEEN BLESSED with a few good mentors. Their finger-prints are present in every insight and absent in every oversight of this book. Their curiosity drove mine, and I hope to convey its full force to my own students and readers. Lawrence D. H. Wood, MD, PhD, of the University of Chicago; John B. West, MD, PhD, DSc, James W. Covell, MD, Richard S. Kornbluth, MD, PhD, and Douglas D. Richman of the University of California, San Diego; and Warren M. Zapol, MD, of Massachusetts General Hospital and Solomon Snyder, MD, DSc, of The Johns Hopkins University taught me to think like a physiologist. In return, I taught them to be patient and persevering.

I am indebted to Sarah Flannery, whose charming book *In Code* reminded me of some long-forgotten brain teasers and also taught me some new ones. I only hope that these little logic puzzles stir my own readers to, like me, stare absently past companions while trying to solve riddles in the middle of the day. These puzzles are a delightful addiction, and they teach reasoning well suited to physiology.

Along with the Cleveland Clinic, I hold a patent on an infusion pump that is intended to measure peripheral venous pressure (PVP). I have a great deal to say about PVP in this book for other reasons, and to teach other lessons, but I do not mention or advocate the use of this specific device.

Finally, I would like to acknowledge the excellent professionals in Mayo Clinic Scientific Publications and Media Support Services who brought this book to life. They include my editor, June Oshiro, PhD, my illustrator, James Tidwell, and the project coordinators who made it all happen: Kenna Atherton, Roberta Schwartz, and LeAnn Stee. Barb Golenzer, our editorial assistant, and John Hedlund, our proofreader, kept us all on the same page. Special thanks go to Joseph G. Murphy, MD, of Mayo Clinic Scientific Press and Doris K. Cope, MD, of the University of Pittsburgh for thinking outside of the box to champion the cause of *Just Enough Physiology*.

CONTENTS

1. Pressure and Its Measurement   1

2. Atmospheric and Alveolar Pressures   12

3. Hydrostatic Pressure   19

4. Doctor Dolittle Visits a Sitting Case   27

5. In the Loop—Left Ventricular Pressures   42

6. What Goes Around Comes Around—Venous Return   48

7. Pushmi-Pullyu and the Right Atrium   55

8. Pressure and Flow—Chickens and Eggs   63

9. Down But Not Out—Circulatory Arrest Pressures   70

10. Starling's Riddle of the Broken Heart   77

11. Oxygen and the Gradients of Life   88

12. The Two Doctors Fick   94

13. A Breath of Fresh Air—Ventilation   101

14. Pulmonary Function Tests   108

15. Where Breath Meets Blood—Lung Perfusion   122

16. Bird Brains and Bird Breath   129

17. Diffusion Limitation—Montana Style   135

18. Man, Machine, and Homeostasis   141

19. Putting It All Together—Manned Space Flight   149

INDEX   157

PRESSURE AND ITS MEASUREMENT

Definition of Pressure

IN PHYSIOLOGIC TERMS, WE are exposed to 3 main sources of pressure: 1) the weight of the atmosphere; 2) hydrostatic forces exerted by the weight of body fluids; and 3) mechanical pressure generated by the heart or other muscles that contract around those fluids. Because cardiopulmonary physiology deals so much with pressure measurements, let's start by defining what pressure really is. Simply put, pressure is force divided by area.

It's also important to understand what pressure is *not*. For example, pressure is not energy. Only when pressure is coupled to a volume change (ie, movement or pressure-volume *work*) is it a component of energy. This is more than just a semantic point. Although we're fond of saying that fluids move from high to low pressure, that isn't always true. The reason why highlights a fundamental difference between pressure and energy. For example, in Figure 1.1, the pipe contains a fluid that is flowing from left to right through a constricted region. The vertical tube in each segment is a pressure manometer.

The eighteenth-century Swiss mathematician Daniel Bernoulli taught us that a fluid in motion contains a total quantity of energy, termed *total fluid energy*. Total fluid energy is simply the sum of 3 elements: 1) pressure energy, a form of potential energy available to push fluid out from the tube if a hole is placed in its wall; 2) hydrostatic

Fluid moves from high to low *total fluid energy*,
not necessarily from high to low *pressure*
Pressure ≠ Energy

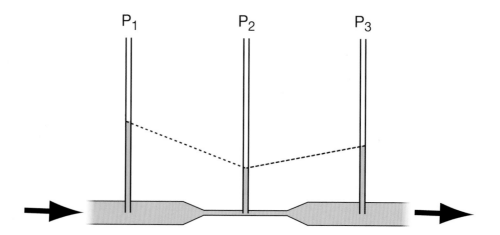

Figure 1.1.   Water Flows Through a Constricted Region.

energy, the potential energy due to elevation of the fluid above a reference point; and 3) kinetic energy of motion.

Total Fluid Energy (per unit of volume) = P + $\rho g z$ + 1/2 ρv^2

where P indicates pressure energy; ρ, density of the fluid; g, acceleration due to gravity; z, height above a reference point; and v, fluid
velocity.

As the fluid moves through the constricted area, it gains speed
(just like a rapid in a narrowing river). More speed means more
kinetic energy. By the law of conservation of energy, the increase
in kinetic energy must be counterbalanced by a decrease in pressure energy; thus, in our example, the pressure manometer in the
narrower segment shows a lower pressure. The law also explains
why the fluid can move from an area of lower pressure (P_2) to
an area of higher pressure (P_3)—that is, because total fluid energy
remains constant (neglecting energy lost through frictional heat).
This application of the law of conservation of energy, widely

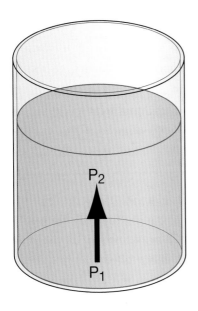

Q: Since $P_1 > P_2$, why doesn't water flow from P_1 to P_2?

A: Because the *total fluid energy* of P_1 = *total fluid energy* of P_2

Figure 1.2. Pressure in a Glass of Water.

known as the *Bernoulli principle*, also pertains to airflow over a wing.

An even simpler example illustrating that fluids do not always move from high to low pressure comes from the physiologist A.C. Burton in his book *Physiology and Biophysics of the Circulation*. In Figure 1.2, the water at the bottom of the glass has a higher pressure than the water at the top, but we know that water doesn't flow spontaneously along the pressure gradient from bottom to top.

The reason is the same as before: the total fluid energy, which includes pressure energy and the energy of position, is the same at the bottom of the glass as it is at the top. P_1 has greater pressure energy than P_2, but P_2 has more energy of position than P_1—and the 2 offset each other exactly.

Let's take another case that's a bit closer to home to see whether you understand the distinction between pressure and energy. Is it accurate to say that the heart generates a pressure gradient that drives blood flow through a resistance? The answer is no. When the heart contracts and generates a pressure gradient, the gradient is abolished as soon as blood flows from one place in the circulation to another. The heart needs to contract again to maintain the difference in total fluid energy between the arteries and veins. The business of the heart is not to maintain pressure gradients—it is to impart fluid energy, which includes a kinetic energy component, to the blood, thereby moving blood from veins to arteries. Pressure gradients are a consequence, not the cause, of that movement of blood. You'll learn more about this in Chapter 8 (Pressure and Flow—Chickens and Eggs).

For the time being, though, consider what happens when we temporarily replace the heart with a mechanical cardiopulmonary bypass system. (It's always instructive to learn from the experience of replacing the function of a normal organ with a mechanical analogue. When we do that, we learn more about the physiology of the natural organ.) Which do we adjust on the machine, pressure or flow? If you didn't know anything else about how cardiopulmonary bypass works, would you say that the machine generates flow and that the pressure gradients observed are the result? Or would you say that the machine generates pressure and flow results? In Chapter 8 (Pressure and Flow—Chickens and Eggs), you'll see the rationale for adopting the former rather than the latter statement.

Measuring Pressure

Pressure is surprisingly difficult to measure. Often, when we think we are measuring pressure, we are actually measuring stretch or movement. A pressure transducer contains a small strain gauge that stretches (or otherwise deforms) in proportion to the pressure difference between the 2 sides. This stretch is coupled to an electrical signal, which is converted to a pressure reading that is referenced ("zeroed") against atmospheric pressure.

The carotid sinus and aortic arch baroreceptors operate with a similar mechanism. Although "baro" means pressure (see the discussion of Mr Torricelli below), these receptors don't measure pressure directly—instead, they measure stretch. In a classic experiment, the carotid sinuses of an anesthetized dog were encased in plaster of Paris while the activity of the carotid sinus nerve ending was recorded. The firing rate did not change with an increase in carotid artery pressure. Only when the sinuses were free to stretch did the carotid artery pressure become coupled to the firing rate of the baroreceptor. This is an important point. All measurements require some exchange of energy; remember, pressure by itself is not energy. In the absence of some volume change or movement, pressure itself cannot generate or give up energy and be measured.

When we monitor hemodynamic properties with invasive lines and pressure transducers, we are actually monitoring very small exchanges of fluid between the patient and the pressure tubing. These volume movements are translated into pressure measurements. The body does the same translation. The autonomic nervous system doesn't know about pressure directly—instead, it knows about how much or how little the baroreceptor walls are being stretched. In other words, it knows about how much blood is being moved from one part of the cardiovascular system to another. We insist on translating this movement into terms of "pressure," but the body doesn't need to speak that language to regulate the cardiovascular system.

When the cardiovascular system responds to a change in stretch, it changes the degree of tension in the vessel walls (through vasoconstriction or vasodilation) and changes the amount of blood that the heart displaces from the veins into the arteries (by changing inotropy or heart rate). In other words, the body senses stretch and responds by changing stretch. Pressure is a somewhat translated and secondary effect of the primary business of the heart, which is to move blood.

You should get a sense from the discussion so far that pressure is a slippery entity. First of all, it is frequently mistaken for energy, but it's not the same; by itself, pressure can move nothing and can perform no work. Second, when we think we're measuring pressure, we're actually measuring something else—the effect of fluid energy, of which pressure is only 1 component. This last point is more technical than practical, though. There's not much harm done in measuring fluid translocation or strain gauge deformation and talking as if we're measuring pressure itself. For all practical and clinical purposes, the distinction doesn't matter. When we get to concepts of venous return and cardiac output, though, you'll see how the mistaken notion that pressure gradients inherently drive blood flow can get you into trouble.

The measurement of pressure brings us back more than 3 and a half centuries to Evangelista Torricelli (Figure 1.3). Torricelli was a remarkable man who served as Galileo's secretary from 1641 to 1642. In 1643, his own assistant, Vincenzo Viviani, used Torricelli's ideas to construct the world's first barometer ("pressure meter" [Figure 1.4]). Viviani filled a tube that was closed on one end with mercury and inverted the tube in a basin of mercury. He noted that the meniscus fell away from the sealed top but did not fall all the way to the bottom—that is, a certain amount of mercury remained in a standing column within the tube, sustained by the vacuum above and by atmospheric pressure below. Torricelli's notion was that the atmosphere itself exerted pressure; therefore, the height of a mercury column below a vacuum should be proportional to atmospheric pressure. This remarkable insight was neither shared nor endorsed by Galileo before the experiment—it was one of the few times where Galileo's intuition failed him.

To further support Torricelli's ideas about the atmosphere exerting pressure, his barometer was taken high into the Italian Alps, where the mercury column was observed to fall, as predicted. This

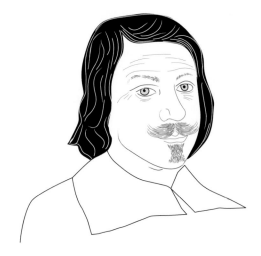

Figure 1.3. Evangelista Torricelli.

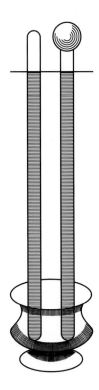

Figure 1.4. Early Mercury Barometer.

(Adapted from Opere dei Discepoli di Galileo, Florence, 1975, as drawn from Torricelli's Letter of June 11 1664 to M. Ricci. Evangelista Torricelli. Scientific career: the barometric experiment [Internet]. Florence [Italy]: Institute and Museum of History of Science; [cited 2010 Nov 15]. Available from: http://www.imss.fi.it/multi/torricel/etorat34.html.)

was not the first demonstration of the variation of barometric pressure with elevation, however; that honor belongs to Florence Périer, the brother-in-law of another great mathematician and scientist, Blaise Pascal. Périer took a barometer up an extinct volcano, the Puy de Dôme in central France, where the meniscus was observed to drop slightly, thereby confirming Torricelli's hypothesis.

The barometer in Figure 1.4 is based on a drawing by Torricelli in a letter to Michelangelo Ricci, the mathematician to the Grand Duke of Florence. In that letter, dated June 11, 1644, Torricelli refuted the belief that "Nature abhors a vacuum." He had actually demonstrated the scientific world's first sustained vacuum and used it to measure the pressure exerted by the atmosphere.

One atmosphere of pressure will sustain a column of mercury that is 760 mm tall (Figure 1.5). In honor of Torricelli, a millimeter of mercury (mm Hg) is also called a Torr. We typically measure pressure in millimeters of mercury or in centimeters of water. Although we use the terms almost interchangeably in medicine, 1 mm Hg is equivalent to 1.36 cm H_2O. The substitution of mercury for water allows an approximate 13-fold decrease in the height of a barometer (Figure 1.6), which makes the device a lot less cumbersome.

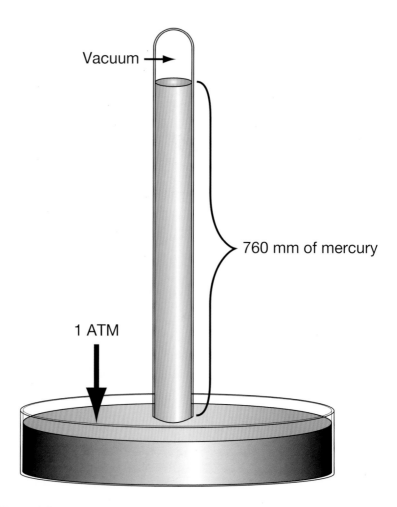

Vacuum

760 mm of mercury

1 ATM

Figure 1.5. Basic Barometer.

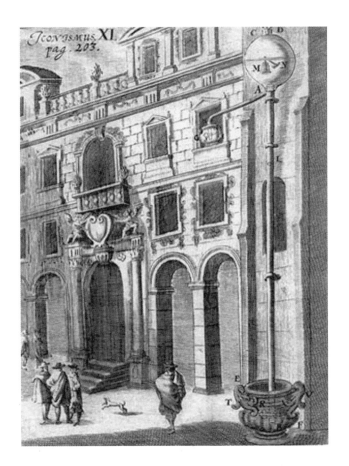

Figure 1.6. Early Water Barometer.

(Adapted from Schott G. Experiment by Gaspare Berti in the Minim Convent
at Pincio [engraving]. Technica curiosa, sive, Mirabilia artis, Würzburg 1664
[Internet]. Florence [Italy]: Institute and Museum of History of Science;
[cited 2010 Nov 15]. Available from: http://www.imss.fi.it/vuoto/eberti.html.)

QUESTIONS AND ANSWERS

Questions

1.1 What is the relationship between pressure and energy? Are they the same thing? Which of the 2 moves blood?

1.2 By the law of conservation of energy, all of the pressure-volume work performed by the heart must be accounted for, but the entire blood volume ends up re-entering back where it started—therefore, no net pressure-volume work is performed. Where does all of that energy go?

1.3 Cite an example of a measurement that requires absolutely no exchange of energy to be performed.

Extra credit A farmer is walking along a road carrying 3 burdens: a goose, a sheaf of wheat, and a fox. He comes to a bridge that can support only his weight plus 1 of the burdens. He can't leave the goose alone with the wheat because the goose will eat the wheat. Similarly, he can't leave the fox and the goose alone together. The fox, however, has no interest in the wheat. How does the farmer get all 3 burdens across?

Answers

1.1 Pressure and energy are not the same. Mathematically, energy is the product of pressure and a volume change ($E = P \times \Delta V$). Physiologically, energy must be added to blood for it to move from one place in the cardiovascular system to another; pressure alone does not necessarily correspond to movement. For example, in a sealed container, pressure can be applied to fluid without the fluid moving. In that circumstance, no work has been performed and no energy has been exchanged. Similarly, water at the bottom of the sea is under high pressure, but it does not necessarily move. Any movement would be attributable to energy (eg, a thermal gradient) being applied, not exposure to high pressure.

1.2 The pressure-volume work of the heart is lost through frictional heat.

1.3 This is a trick question. All physiologic measurements require an exchange of energy. For example, a change in blood pressure is detected by observing movement of a fluid meniscus, a deformation of a strain gauge diaphragm, or the compression and release of an artery beneath a blood pressure cuff. Each of these methods of measurement involves movement, and all movements involve an exchange of energy.

Extra credit The farmer leaves the fox and wheat behind while walking the goose across. Then he returns for the fox. After he carries the fox across, he leaves it alone while returning with the goose. He leaves the goose on the original side while crossing with the wheat. He then leaves the fox and wheat together on the far side and returns for the goose.

ATMOSPHERIC AND ALVEOLAR PRESSURES

NOW THAT YOU KNOW what pressure is and how it's measured, let's apply what you know to human physiology. Memorizing respiratory physiology equations out of context, though, is like having a root canal: it's good for you, but it's hardly welcoming. That's why we're going to put respiration in a more interesting context.

First, a few nomenclature items to take care of: "P" denotes pressure, of course (measured in mm Hg or torr, unless otherwise noted). Small capital "A" denotes alveolar. Lowercase "a" represents arterial. "P_B" is barometric pressure. "R" is the respiratory quotient, which is simply the ratio of CO_2 produced by the body divided by the amount of O_2 consumed. "P_{H_2O}" is the vapor pressure of water. F_{IO_2} is the fraction of inspired O_2, with 1.0 equivalent to 100% inspired oxygen. P_{IO_2} is the partial pressure of inspired oxygen.

In 1978, 2 climbers (Reinhold Messner and Peter Habeler) reached the summit of Mount Everest (Figure 2.1) without using supplemental oxygen. Physiologists originally thought such a climb was impossible because a calculation of lung oxygen levels at that altitude indicated that nothing beyond basal metabolism could be supported, even with hyperventilation. Thus, a climber theoretically would not have sufficient oxygen available for the exercise that was needed to reach the summit in the first place.

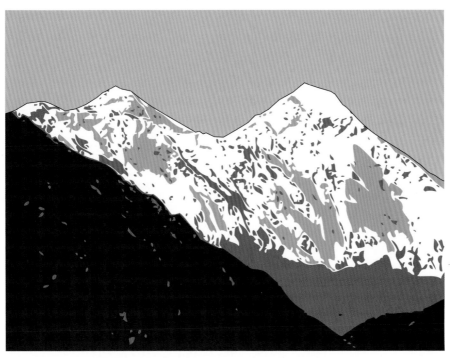

Mount Everest
Summit = 8,848 m (29,028 ft)
P_B = 253 mm Hg
pH of arterial blood = 7.7
P_{ACO_2} = 7 mm Hg
P_{AO_2} = 35 mm Hg
Pa_{O_2} = 28 mm Hg

Figure 2.1.   Mount Everest.

P_B denotes barometric pressure; P_{ACO_2}, alveolar carbon dioxide pressure; P_{AO_2}, alveolar oxygen pressure; Pa_{O_2}, arterial oxygen pressure.

When Messner and Habeler proved the physiologists wrong, it was time for the scientists to go back to the drawing board. For the enterprising Dr. John West, an international authority in high-altitude physiology and medicine, this meant going back to Everest. He had already accompanied a scientific expedition there in the early 1960s, but very little physiologic data were available from that (or subsequent) expeditions. In October 1981, 5 climbers made it to the summit of Everest. There, West and a team of physicians and physiologists took the first careful atmospheric and physiologic measurements from the summit.

As you might expect, what they found was interesting. First, the atmospheric pressure was higher than that predicted by the International Civil Aviation Organization charts, which plot estimated pressure against altitude. The reason for the discrepancy is because barometric pressure is affected by latitude, as well as by altitude. A dense, cold air mass is present in the stratosphere at low latitudes, and Everest is at relatively low latitude. Second, researchers were surprised by the degree of alveolar and arterial gas abnormalities, which you can review in Figure 2.1.

Now, back down to the ground. What you need to know, either to study altitude physiology or to monitor patients in the operating room or intensive care unit, is how to calculate alveolar oxygen pressure (P_{AO_2}) and how to compare that calculated value with the measured arterial oxygen pressure (Pa_{O_2}). This difference (P_{AO_2}–Pa_{O_2}), also termed AaD_{O_2}, gives an estimate of how efficiently the lungs are oxygenating the blood. There are several physiologic causes of hypoxemia (Box 2.1). Hypoventilation, lowered P_{IO_2}, and lowered P_B will not increase AaD_{O_2}. The other 3 will.

How do we estimate P_{AO_2}? There is a relatively simple equation, the "alveolar air equation," that accomplishes this. It is worth memorizing because you'll use it again and again:

$$P_{AO_2} = \underbrace{(P_B - P_{H_2O})\,F_{IO_2}}_{P_{IO_2}} - (P_{ACO_2}/R)$$

We have already defined each of the terms. You should note that the equation is frequently misrepresented, with "Pa_{CO_2}" (instead of "P_{ACO_2}") in the numerator of the second term. We often substitute the arterial P_{CO_2} for alveolar P_{CO_2} when making

Box 2.1. Physiologic Causes of Hypoxemia

Causes alveolar-arterial gradient
    Diffusion impairment
    Ventilation/perfusion (V/Q) mismatch
    Shunt
Does not cause alveolar-arterial gradient
    Hypoventilation
    Lowered F_{IO_2}
    Lowered P_B

the calculation for a specific patient, and since there isn't usually much of a CO_2 gradient across the lung, it doesn't make a lot of difference. Nevertheless, be aware that the real equation uses the alveolar value (remember, this is the *alveolar* air equation), rather than the arterial value for CO_2.

Now that you know this equation, plug in the actual values from the summit of Everest (Figure 2.1). Use a value of 0.8 for R. (R=1.0 if you eat only carbohydrates, R=0.7 if you eat only fats, and R=0.8 for a mixed diet or if you eat only protein.) Use a value of 47 mm Hg for P_{H_2O}. You'll notice that if the climber *didn't* massively hyperventilate (P_{ACO_2} = 7 mm Hg!), his alveolar P_{O_2} would be even lower than 35 mm Hg. For reference, a normal P_{aO_2} at sea level is 100 mm Hg, and P_{ACO_2} when ventilating normally is 40 mm Hg.

How can an alveolar P_{O_2} of 35 mm Hg and an arterial P_{O_2} of 28 mm Hg be compatible with life and exercise? What other aspect of the blood gas gives you a hint? What oxygen saturation would you expect with this blood gas if there *wasn't* a leftward shift in the oxyhemoglobin dissociation curve (Figure 2.2)? What is this subject's AaD_{O_2}? (Extra-extra credit: why is there an AaD_{O_2} at all in this unusually fit subject? If you can guess the answer to that, the coffee is on me. If not, the answer is in Chapter 17, Diffusion Limitation—Montana Style).

One aspect of the alveolar air equation that may not be apparent is the role of P_{H_2O}. Remember that water vapor is just that—a vapor, not a gas. At body temperature, P_{H_2O} is 47 mm Hg. That means that if the atmospheric pressure was only 47 mm Hg and the atmosphere was completely saturated with water vapor at 37°C, there would be no room left for atmospheric gases. Therefore, the partial pressure of actual lung gases make up the fraction of the total pressure remaining after water vapor pressure is taken into account.

There is one other thing about atmospheric pressure that you should know—the F_{IO_2} remains essentially unchanged (value, 0.21) as altitude increases, although the P_{IO_2} changes. It's useful to memorize a simplified alveolar air equation for patients who are breathing ambient (room) air at sea level. What is that P_{IO_2}?

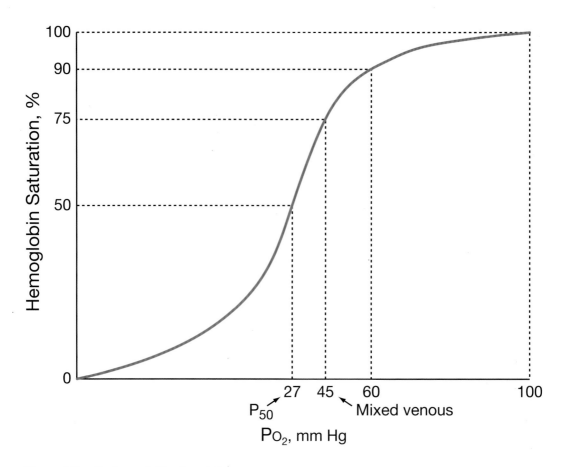

Figure 2.2. Oxyhemoglobin dissociation curve.

P_{50} is the partial pressure of oxygen at which 50% of the hemoglobin is saturated.

QUESTIONS AND ANSWERS

Questions

2.1 Write out the alveolar air equation from memory and describe each component.

2.2 Solve the alveolar air equation for a subject breathing ambient air at sea level, with P_{ACO_2} = 40 mm Hg, and eating only carbohydrates.

2.3 Solve the alveolar air equation for a subject breathing ambient air on the summit of Mount Everest, but with P_{ACO_2} = 20 mm Hg and eating only fats.

2.4 In the alveolar air equation, why is water vapor pressure (P_{H_2O}) subtracted from atmospheric pressure (P_B) when calculating P_{AO_2}?

Extra credit You are in the basement of a house and are looking at 3 adjacent light switches, all in the "off" position. Only one of those switches is connected to an incandescent bulb in the attic, which you can't see from the basement. You are allowed to manipulate 2 of the switches and are allowed to make only 1 trip to the attic. How can you determine which of the 3 switches is connected to the light?

Answers

2.1 $P_{AO_2} = (P_B - P_{H_2O})F_{IO_2} - (P_{ACO_2}/R)$

Each term is defined in the chapter. Remember that water vapor pressure (P_{H_2O}) is temperature dependent, and that at body temperature, it is 47 mm Hg. This is an equation that is used often and worth memorizing.

2.2 $P_{AO_2} = (760 - 47)0.21 - (40/1) = 109.7$ mm Hg

2.3 $P_{AO_2} = (253 - 47)0.21 - (20/0.7) = 14.7$ mm Hg.

This alveolar oxygen level is incompatible with life!

2.4 Water vapor excludes dry gases; thus, the partial pressure of water vapor lowers the partial pressure contributions of dry gases in the atmosphere.

Extra credit Turn one of the switches to the "on" position for 5 minutes and then switch it off. Turn the next switch to the "on" position and leave it on. Go up to the attic. If the light is on, it is connected to the second switch. If it is off but hot to the touch, it is connected to the first switch. If it is off but cool, it is connected to the third switch.

HYDROSTATIC PRESSURE

HERE'S WHERE PRESSURE GETS interesting—in fact, counterintuitive. If you're going to understand how to think about pressures within the circulatory system, though, you'll need to know a few of the not-so-obvious principles of hydrostatics. Take the example illustrated in Figure 3.1. This cartoon is meant to emphasize the point that hydrostatic pressure depends only on the vertical distance of the fluid, not on the shape of its container. The medical student at the bottom of a cone-shaped pool experiences the same pressure as the student at the bottom of a cylindrical pool (Figure 3.1A). The "extra" water above and on the sides of the student in the cone does not contribute to the hydrostatic pressure at the bottom. Again, only the vertical distance matters. If you doubt this, consider Figure 3.1B. If the pressure at the bottom of a conical pool really was higher than that at the bottom of a cylindrical pool (assuming the cone holds more water than the cylinder), we could connect the pools as shown and expect to have a perpetual motion machine. That doesn't happen, of course, because hydrostatic pressure is affected only by the density of the fluid, its vertical height above or below a measurement point, and the acceleration due to gravity.

Now suppose that you still didn't believe and decided to perform an experiment to prove that a large body of fluid has greater pressure beneath it than a smaller body. To do this, you pipe water from

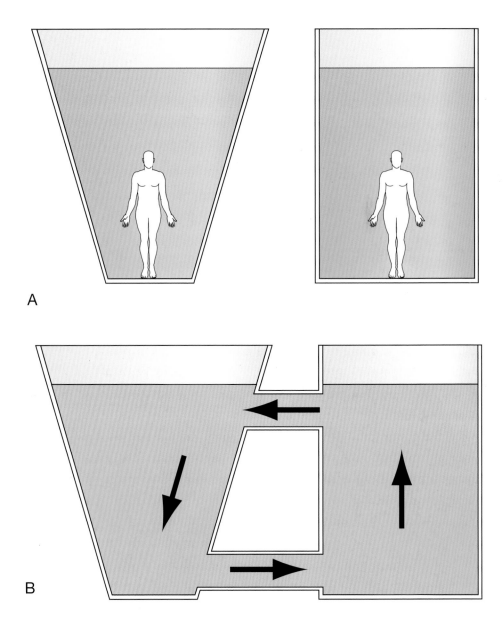

Figure 3.1. A, Medical students at the bottom of a conical pool and a cylindrical pool. B, A perpetual motion machine?

a hole drilled near the bottom of the Atlantic Ocean through a vertical pipe that emerges next to your house (Figure 3.2). If the larger mass of water in the ocean exerts greater pressure than the smaller mass of water in your vertical pipe, then you should see water perpetually flowing through the pipe and rising higher than sea level.

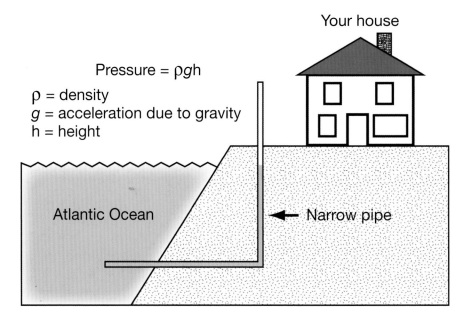

Figure 3.2. Does a large body of water have greater pressure beneath it than a small body of water?

Could you then tap into this continual flow with a water wheel to generate energy? Of course not.

Continual flow doesn't happen in this example for the same reason as described above—hydrostatic pressure is not determined by the shape of the fluid container or the total mass of fluid that it contains. Here, only the vertical distance above the measurement point is important. This concept is basically a restatement of *Pascal's Principle*, which holds that pressure is equally distributed throughout a continuous fluid—*at the same vertical level*.

Now let's apply these principles to the siphon, defined as any fluid-filled conduit that excludes air. The reason for broaching this issue is that the cardiovascular system also obeys the principle of the siphon. A simple siphon is depicted in Figure 3.3. The portion of the siphon that is above the upper reservoir has negative transmural pressure and will suck air in if it is perforated (like a venous sinus in a sitting craniotomy). That's why air embolism can occur when the operative site is above the level of the heart, even when the patient is being mechanically ventilated and has only above-atmospheric

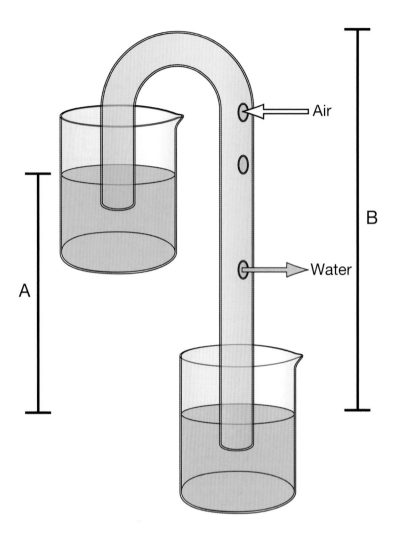

Figure 3.3. Simple Siphon.

pressures in the chest. The portion of the siphon below the level of the upper reservoir will have positive transmural pressure and will expel fluid if perforated. *Transmural pressure* is the pressure inside a vessel minus the pressure outside. Don't confuse transmural pressure with *perfusion pressure*, which is inlet minus outlet pressure.

Let's see if you understand these principles so far. What is the perfusion pressure in Figure 3.3—ρgA or ρgB? If we leave the 2 water baths at the same level but extend the upper loop of the siphon (ie, increase its height), will the transmural pressure at the top change? If so, in what direction? Will the perfusion pressure of the system change? Will the resistance change? Will the flow change? If the flow changes, is it because the resistance has changed or because the perfusion pressure has changed? (The answers to these questions are at the end of this chapter.)*

Let's take a more complicated siphon and apply virtually all of the principles that you've just learned. If you understand this, you will understand the physics involved in air embolism in sitting or prone patients. Figure 3.4 shows 2 siphons (inverted U-shaped tubes) filled with water. Just like water doesn't drain from a straw capped by a finger, water does not drain out of either limb of either siphon. One may intuitively think that the lesser mass of water in the thin limb of siphon A can't possibly counterbalance the greater mass of water in the thick limb, but that in fact isn't true. A siphon can have

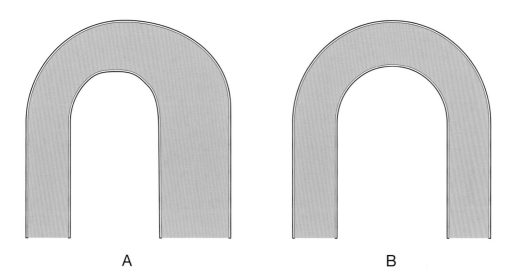

A   B

Figure 3.4.   Siphons With Limbs of Unequal Diameter.

---

* Answers to the siphon questions: 1) The perfusion pressure is "A," not "B." Remember, the perfusion pressure of an enclosed fluid path is simply inlet minus outlet pressures, and the route between the 2 does not matter. 2) Yes, the transmural pressure (the inside minus the outside pressure at that point) at the top of a siphon limb will decrease if the limb is made higher, but the perfusion pressure (inlet minus outlet pressure) will remain the same. 3) The resistance will change because the length of tubing increases (see Poiseuille's Law in Chapter 4). 4) The flow will decrease as a result of increased resistance, not because of a change in perfusion pressure, because perfusion pressure does not change.

limbs of unequal diameter or shape and still function just the same. Why is that? The reason is that a siphon balances the pressure, not the fluid mass, of its 2 limbs. Remember that pressure is simply the product of fluid density, height of the fluid column above or below a reference point, and acceleration due to gravity. Total fluid mass is not a component of pressure.

The Romans understood the principles of the siphon very well. They were able to construct aqueducts that brought water through deep valleys without having to always build bridges like the one shown in Figure 3.5. To accomplish this, they extended siphons (inverted U-shaped conduits) down one side of the valley and back up the other side to a point that was slightly lower than the starting point.

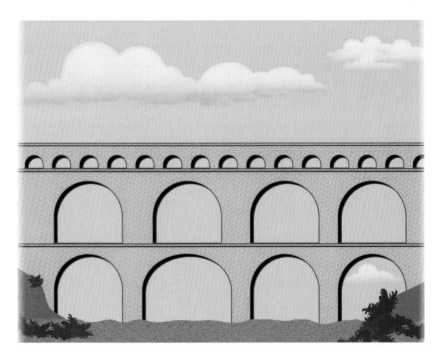

Figure 3.5. Roman Aqueduct Bridge.

QUESTIONS AND ANSWERS

Questions

3.1 What is the difference between transmural pressure and perfusion pressure?

3.2 Is there a relationship between transmural pressure, which can vary at different points within a fluid circuit, and flow through that circuit?

3.3 Will the presence of 1-way valves that open downward affect the hydrostatic pressure measured at the bottom of a vessel that contains such valves?

3.4 A "friend" has talked you into a combined scuba-diving and spelunking adventure. You dive to a depth of 30 feet before entering a submerged cave. After entering the cave, you swim exactly 10 feet up, 40 feet down, then 30 feet back up through a complicated series of tunnels and underwater caverns before coming to rest in a channel that is exactly 30 feet below sea level. What is your pressure gauge reading now? What principle have you invoked in answering this question?

Extra credit A traveler arrives at a remote inn and asks the surly proprietor for a room for 7 nights. The traveler has no money, he has only 7 gold rings linked together in a linear chain. The innkeeper demands payment of 1 gold ring per night. The traveler knows better than to hand over the whole chain ahead of time and agrees only to pay as he goes—one ring per night, even though that will mean cutting the chain. The innkeeper states that cut rings aren't as valuable as intact rings. The traveler devises a way of paying what he owes as he goes. What is the minimal number of cuts that he can make to accomplish this?

Answers

3.1 Transmural pressure, which means "across the wall," is the difference between the pressure on the inside of a vessel and the pressure on the outside of the vessel at the same place. Perfusion pressure is the difference between pressure at the inlet of a vessel and pressure at the outlet.

3.2 No. Transmural pressure does not affect blood flow. (Blood flow correlates with perfusion pressure.)

3.3 No. A 1-way valve allowing downward flow will not protect what's below it from the pressure above it.

3.4 The pressure is equivalent to 30 feet of sea water (approximately 1 atmosphere above barometric pressure at sea level). The path taken between 2 points in a continuous body of fluid is irrelevant. Pressure is determined only by fluid density (ρ), acceleration due to gravity (g) and height relative to a reference point (h). In this case, the reference point is sea level and depth is 30 feet at both locations. This is another application of Pascal's Principle (pressure is equally distributed throughout a continuous fluid at the same vertical level).

Extra credit One cut. This is made though the third ring in the chain of 7. On the first night, the traveler gives the innkeeper the cut ring. On the second night, he asks for the cut ring back and gives the innkeeper the chain of 2 rings (rings 1 and 2 in the original chain). On the third night, he adds the cut ring to the other 2. On night 4, he retrieves the 3 rings and gives the innkeeper the uncut chain of 4. On night 5, he adds the cut ring back. On night 6, he retrieves the cut ring and adds the chain of 2. On the last night, he adds back the cut ring.

· 4 ·

DOCTOR DOLITTLE VISITS
A SITTING CASE

IF YOU THINK YOU understand the circulatory system, test yourself by studying the giraffe (Figure 4.1). This mysterious animal has preoccupied some of the world's best physiologists and has engendered a bit of controversy along the way. It all started with the observation that the giraffe's blood pressure is quite high, approximately 250 mm Hg (systolic). The obvious explanation for this pressure is that the towering giant has to pump blood "so far uphill" to its head. As with so many other principles in hemodynamics, however, the common-sense answer fails us and the correct answer is more complicated.

Let's start off by considering that the giraffe isn't always a "heads-up" creature. When it leans over to drink water, for example, the head is much lower than the heart (Figure 4.2). That raises the following question: if the giraffe has such high blood pressure to compensate for gravity when its head is elevated, what happens when its head is down? Does the blood pressure fall below normal to compensate in the opposite direction? Before engaging in the details of circulatory physiology in these unusual animals, let's cut to the chase with the final answer: the giraffe does not have to compensate for gravity in either circumstance. When the head is down, the heart pumps blood downhill, of course, but it also has to pump the venous blood uphill. Ultimately, gravity neither helps nor hinders

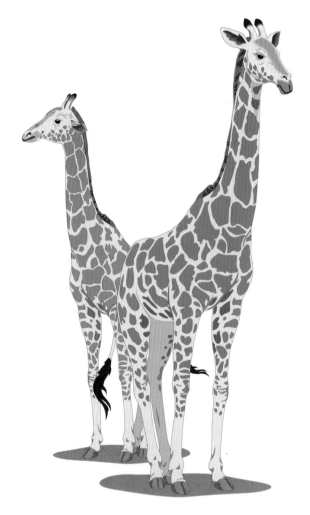

Figure 4.1. Giraffes.

the total blood flow to the head, and gravity need not be considered in calculating perfusion pressure or flow.

This may be intuitive for the case of a head-down animal, but it doesn't seem to be intuitive for most people when they consider the head-up animal. Nonetheless, the same answer holds in both circumstances—the heart has to pump blood uphill to the head when the giraffe is standing, and it also receives venous blood flowing downhill to the heart. How does downhill venous return help uphill arterial flow? If the venous blood were in free fall, like a waterfall in open air, it wouldn't help—but the venous blood isn't in free fall. It is contained within the tubing of the vascular system, and any time

A

B

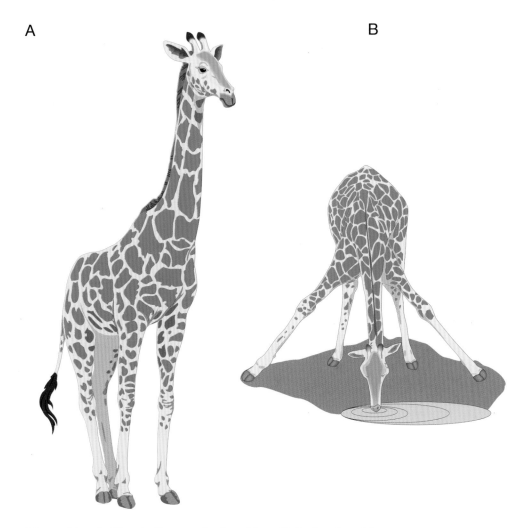

Figure 4.2. A, The giraffe not only does this… B, It also does this.

fluid flows through tubing that excludes air, siphon principles apply. In this section, you'll learn more about siphons than you ever cared to, but that's what Dr Dolittle calls for if you're to understand either standing giraffes or patients undergoing sitting craniotomies.

Any explanation for the cerebral circulation of giraffes must not only be robust enough to contend with different head positions, but it must also explain data obtained from direct measurement of jugular venous pressure in the animals. An acceptable model must also explain why the cerebral circulation continues to work in weightless environments (ie, during space flight). Finally, it must explain the clinical phenomenon of air embolism, which is what happens when air gets sucked into perforated veins or sinuses when the surgical site is above the heart.

I'm going to show you 2 models of the cerebral circulation: the first is a common-sense model that most of us would draw without having thought about it much; the second is a model that makes a lot more physical sense and answers the questions above in a way that the first model cannot. The main difference between these models is that the correct one takes into account the principle of the siphon, whereas the incorrect one does not.

Let's go back to the giraffe. The pressures measured at different points in the jugular vein are not at all what you would expect. When the right atrial pressure is measured in the standing, sedated giraffe, it is lower than expected—that is, it is lower than the pressure in a standing column of blood the same height as a giraffe's neck. This paradox is not confined only to exotic African animals. Patients in the sitting position demonstrate the same phenomenon. For example, let's say that the tip of a central venous pressure (CVP) catheter is at the junction between the superior vena cava and the right atrium, the pressure transducer is at the level of the heart, and the head is elevated such that the vertical distance between the top of the head (superior sagittal sinus) and the heart is 25 cm. You notice that the CVP registers a pressure equivalent to 2 to 3 cm H_2O. How can that happen? As I alluded to before, it happens because of the siphon effect, which you'll read about below—but first, let's look at the data from physiologist Henry Badeer's intriguing study of hemodynamic properties of the giraffe jugular vein.

Dr Badeer placed a very long CVP catheter down the jugular vein from above, while keeping the pressure transducer zeroed and at the level of the head (Figure 4.3). If you did this without a giraffe and just lowered the saline-filled catheter further and further below the transducer in open air, you would notice that the recorded pressure decreased as the catheter tip descended. This occurs because the column of saline in the catheter "pulls down" on the transducer above it and exposes the transducer to suction (ie, negative pressure). Keep that negative pressure in mind because it will explain another paradox about humans who have their heads elevated during

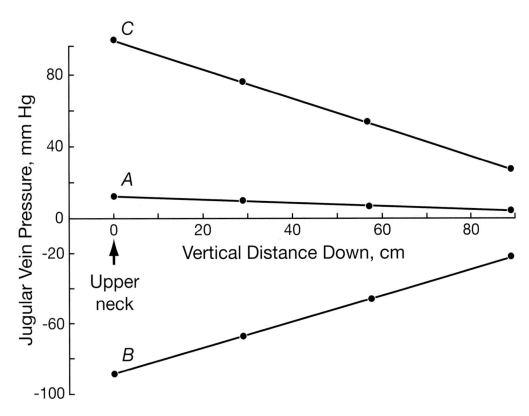

Figure 4.3. Plot of Pressure Components in the Jugular Vein of the Standing, Sedated Giraffe. A, Pressure in the vein. B, Increasing gravitational component of pressure down the vein. C, Decreasing pressure due to viscous resistance to flow. (Adapted from Badeer HS. Haemodynamics of the jugular vein in the giraffe [letter]. Nature. 1988 Apr 28;332[6167]:788-9. Used with permission.)

surgery—that is, how air gets sucked into a punctured vein or a sinus when the head is higher than the heart.

Returning to the giraffe, though—when Dr Badeer lowered his CVP catheter down the giraffe's jugular vein, the pressure measurements recorded by the stationary transducer above remained essentially the same (Figure 4.3, line A). To explain that, the pressure within the vein must have been very low (below atmospheric) at the top and much higher at the bottom. The combination of the vein's pressure getting higher with increasing distance from the head exactly counterbalanced the tendency of the CVP catheter to record lower pressures as it descended, resulting in a reading that stayed virtually the same at all heights.

The only way that pressure in a column of fluid (eg, blood in the jugular vein) could be below atmospheric at the top and essentially atmospheric at the bottom is if it were suspended by suction from above. This is the same as a column of soda in a straw (ie, when you plug the top of a filled straw with your finger and lift the straw out of the bottle), and it also holds true in a siphon. A siphon is any arrangement of fluid-filled tubing that excludes air and is open on both ends to allow flow. If the 2 open ends are at the same height, no flow occurs and no fluid leaks out. If one end is lower than the other, flow starts and continues out the lower end. If the upper end of the siphon is submerged in a container of fluid, it will drain the container.

The siphon in Figure 4.4 further illustrates that pressure at different points in the tubing depends on the height relative to the upper fluid source. Any point in the siphon above the upper fluid source will have negative (subatmospheric) pressure—poke a hole in any part of a siphon above the upper fluid source, and air will get sucked into the hole. In contrast, if you poke a hole in the tubing at any point below the upper fluid source, the fluid below the new hole will fall out of the tubing, displaced by air that enters the tubing just after the hole is made. After this drainage occurs, the fluid from above the hole will leak out of the hole, and the siphon action will continue to drain fluid from the tubing above the hole.

One other thing that you should know about siphons is how to calculate the perfusion pressure. In the same figure, the perfusion pressure is proportional to height "A" (not height "B"). The path that the siphon takes is irrelevant to flow. The relative height between the beginning and end of the circuit is all that matters. If the open ends are at the same level, the 2 limbs of the siphon balance each other and no spontaneous flow occurs. Still, even though no fluid flows, a wide range of "transmural pressures" occur within the siphon. Transmural pressure is simply the difference between the internal and external pressure at a given point. It is not the same as perfusion pressure, and it has nothing to do with flow.

It happens that the cerebral circulation functions like a siphon. That is, like an inverted "U," it constitutes a continuous column of fluid that extends from the heart to the head and back down to the heart again. If you remember our previous discussion about

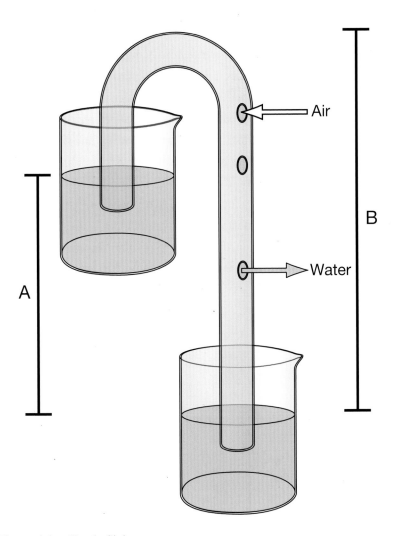

Figure 4.4. Simple Siphon.

hydrostatic pressure, any continuous column of fluid that begins and ends at the same vertical height is gravitationally neutral—fluid won't tend to move in either direction within an inverted U-shaped tube unless it's provided with a mechanical push (by the heart, for instance).

When mechanically ventilated patients are placed in the sitting position, their thoracic pressures are either at atmospheric pressure (end expiration) or above atmospheric pressure (during inspiration). Nonetheless, air can get sucked into punctured cerebral veins or sinuses, and this phenomenon (air embolism) is more likely to happen when the punctured vessel is high above the heart. One property of siphons is that they explain how negative transmural pressure can occur, even in the absence of a vacuum or without a suction source being applied. If the sinuses and veins of the head constitute one limb of a siphon circuit, then we can predict that the highest reaches of that circuit will have subatmospheric pressures and will suck in air if perforated. In contrast, if the cerebral veins are simply dropping blood back down to the heart over a sort of "vascular waterfall," (Figure 4.5, left), then it is impossible to explain air embolism.

A waterfall does not generate negative pressure anywhere along its length. Nor does a waterfall model predict the sorts of pressures that Dr Badeer measured in the giraffe's jugular vein. If you drop a CVP catheter down a waterfall while keeping the transducer at the

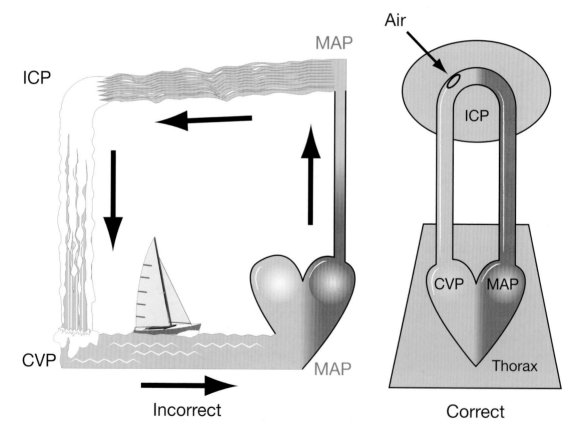

Figure 4.5. Two Models of a Circulatory System.

CVP denotes central venous pressure; ICP, intracranial pressure; MAP, mean arterial pressure. (Adapted from Munis JR, Lozada LJ. Giraffes, siphons, and Starling resistors: cerebral perfusion pressure revisited [editorial]. J Neurosurg Anesthesiol. 2000 Jul;12[3]:290-6. Used with permission.)

top, the recorded pressures will progressively decrease as the catheter tip descends (just as it would in free air). If you understand that the cerebral circulation occurs in a closed circuit (Figure 4.5, right), Dr Badeer's measurements are predicted, the phenomenon of air embolism is explained, and your model is robust enough to describe blood flow to the brain in supine, head-up, and head-down positions, as well as in a weightless environment.

The siphon model of circulation is gravitationally neutral. Because the cerebral circulation begins and ends at the heart level, the path taken between the brain and the heart (up and then down again, down and then up, or always at the same level) doesn't matter. Flow will depend only on the resistance of the tubing and the energy added by the heart to move blood through that resistance.

So the pressure within the superior vena cava in a sitting human or in a standing giraffe is really just the residual mechanical pressure from the heart after being degraded by vascular resistance. It's not the hydrostatic pressure at the bottom of an isolated column of fluid. That's how the CVP reading in a sitting patient can be far less than that suggested by the vertical distance from the top of the head to the heart. That's also how a giraffe's right atrial pressure can be so much lower than expected, given the length of its neck.

Figure 4.6 illustrates the difference between cerebral perfusion pressure and local transmural pressure. At any point in the cerebral circulation, the local transmural pressure (inside minus outside pressure in that segment of vessel) is simply the sum of the mechanical pressure generated by the heart, intracranial pressure, and hydrostatic pressure relative to the heart level. Anatomically, the cerebral circulation may be divided into 4 zones: 1) extracranial arterial; 2) intracranial arterial and venous; 3) intracranial sinus (shielded from intracranial pressure); and 4) extracranial venous. Intracranial pressure exists only within zone 2. Hydrostatic pressure relative to the heart begins and ends at 0 because the cerebral circulation begins and ends at the heart level. Note that this graph depicts pressure in a subject sitting upright—the $\rho g h$ line bows downward to reach a maximal negative pressure midway through the cerebral circulation (sagittal sinus). If the subject was supine, the $\rho g h$ line would be flat and at a constant value of 0 because gravity does not contribute to

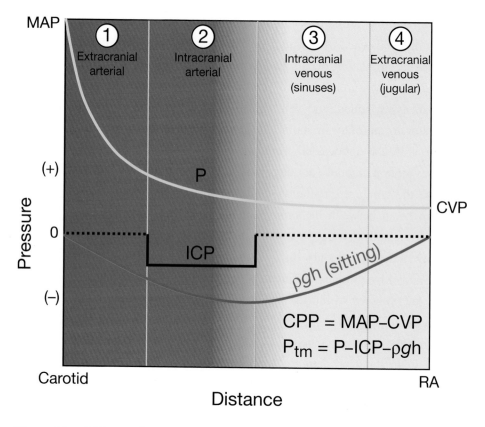

Figure 4.6. Difference Between Cerebral Perfusion Pressure and Local Transmural Pressure.

CPP denotes cerebral perfusion pressure; CVP, central venous pressure; ICP, intracranial pressure; MAP, mean arterial pressure; P, mechanical pressure generated by the heart; P_{tm}, transmural pressure; RA, right atrium; ρgh, hydrostatic pressure relative to the heart level. (Adapted from Munis JR, Lozada LJ. Giraffes, siphons, and Starling resistors: cerebral perfusion pressure revisited [editorial]. J Neurosurg Anesthesiol. 2000 Jul;12[3]:290-6. Used with permission.)

local transmural pressure in the supine position. If the subject was in a head-down position, the ρgh line would bow upward to reach a maximal positive value midway through the cerebral circulation; hydrostatic pressure would contribute positively to transmural pressure at that level.

What about the extraordinarily high blood pressure of the giraffe? Doesn't that have anything to do with having to push blood so far uphill? No—remember the lessons from the siphon and what it means for a fluid path to be gravitationally neutral. This concept is neatly summarized by the physiologist A.C. Burton: "It is no harder, in the circulation, for blood to flow uphill than downhill."

The reason, then, why a giraffe's systolic blood pressure is 250 mm Hg is not because its heart has to push blood so far uphill—it is because it has to push blood through very long carotid arteries. Resistance to laminar flow is directly affected by the length of the tube through which the flow occurs, as illustrated by Poiseuille's Law:

$$Q = K \Delta P \pi r^4 / 8 \eta l$$

where Q indicates flow; K, a constant; ΔP, pressure gradient; r, radius; η, viscosity; and l, length. This means that, everything else being equal, if a giraffe's carotid artery is 3 times as long as a human's, the pressure gradient across it will be 3 times as large at comparable flows.

Put another way, a giraffe doesn't need to modulate its blood pressure upward to compensate for the standing position any more than it needs to modulate it downward to compensate for the head-down position while drinking water. This is because its cerebral circulation is a closed loop—and *cerebral perfusion pressure* is unaffected by gravity, even though *local transmural pressure* is affected by gravity. As the heart generates flow through a high-resistance circulatory system, the resulting pressures will be high, regardless of position.

What about the fact that cerebral blood vessels and jugular veins are collapsible? Doesn't that negate the siphon effect and prevent the downward (venous) part of the circuit from counterbalancing the upward (arterial) part? The answer is no. The blood vessels in the brain are collapsible only in theory. In fact, they are surrounded by the fluid consistency of the brain and by the rigid skull. This isovolumic (constant total volume) system makes it impossible for the cerebral vessels to completely collapse.

You can demonstrate this phenomenon yourself by inflating a balloon with air inside of an iced tea jar with the mouth of the balloon attached to the spigot at the bottom. Fill the jar around the balloon with water and then seal the top of the jar. If you now open the spigot at the bottom, the balloon remains inflated. It can't collapse because the isovolumic jar has no additional water to displace it.

How about the jugular veins and other venous drainage vessels in the neck? They also are collapsible in theory, but collectively, they support 750 mL/min of cerebral venous drainage and are never fully collapsed. If they were to do so, the head would swell. Modeling experiments, including those of the author, have demonstrated that "collapsible" tubing is perfectly capable of supporting siphon drainage, even after it has assumed a partially collapsed shape during flow.

Does this mean that the circulation of the brain operates by siphoning blood through the head? No—remember that the cerebral circulation is a closed loop that begins and ends at the same level (ie, at the heart). Blood circulates through the brain because of the pumping of the heart. The "siphon effect" in this case, with 2 limbs of equal height, doesn't passively siphon blood. Instead, this closed loop arrangement simply maintains gravitational neutrality so that the heart doesn't have to work against gravity. It has to work only against resistance.

Let's put this all together in terms of the giraffe. When the giraffe raises its head, the transmural pressure at the top of the cerebral circuit decreases. When it lowers its head to drink, the transmural pressure at the bottom of the circuit (in the now lowered head) increases. In both cases, however, the perfusion pressure never changes because the perfusion pressure remains mean arterial pressure minus CVP, and those 2 heart-level pressures don't change significantly with head position.

If you understand the difference between transmural pressure and perfusion pressure—congratulations! That distinction has escaped many good minds, which is probably why the anesthesia and monitoring textbooks still make the mistake of recommending that arterial pressure transducer be positioned at the level of the head, rather than the heart, in sitting patients, supposedly to compensate for a reduced perfusion pressure to the elevated head. Moving a pressure transducer upward automatically lowers the reading in proportion to how high you've raised it. Such a maneuver will predict changes in local transmural pressure (which has nothing to do with flow), but doesn't (and can't) tell you anything about the unchanged perfusion pressure.

SUGGESTED READING

Hicks JW, Badeer, HS. Gravity and the circulation: "open" vs. "closed" systems. Am J Physiol. 1992 May;262(5 Pt 2):R725-32.

Hicks JW, Munis JR. The siphon controversy counterpoint: the brain need not be "baffling." Am J Physiol Regul Integr Comp Physiol. 2005 Aug;289(2):R629-32.

Munis JR, Lozada LJ. Giraffes, siphons, and Starling resistors: cerebral perfusion pressure revisited [editorial]. J Neurosurg Anesthesiol. 2000 Jul;12(3):290-6.

QUESTIONS AND ANSWERS

While visiting the San Diego Zoo, you are asked to measure the sagittal sinus pressure in a standing giraffe and to compare the pressure inside the sinus to atmospheric pressure. The difference between them is the transmural pressure of the sinus, and it is an indicator of the tendency of the giraffe toward venous air embolism, should a sinus be perforated and exposed to the atmosphere (something you're careful not to do, of course). You record a pressure of –200 cm H_2O. The head is 200 cm above the heart. The mean arterial blood pressure (measured at the level of the heart) is 250 cm H_2O. To simplify calculations, assume that 1 cm of blood is equivalent to 1 mm Hg of hydrostatic pressure.

Questions

4.1 What would be the mean arterial pressure measured at the head?

4.2 As blood moves from the intracranial arteries through the capillaries and into the intracranial sinuses, how much does the pressure decrease?

4.3 While taking your measurements, the giraffe's heart stops momentarily, and its mean arterial pressure (measured at the level of the heart) decreases to 15 cm H_2O, which is the same as the right atrial pressure both before and after the cardiac arrest. What is the mean arterial pressure now, measured at the level of the head?

4.4 What has happened to the gradient between the intracranial artery and the intracranial sinus?

4.5 Assuming that intracranial pressure is unchanged, what has happened to the cerebral perfusion pressure? Is it a negative number?

4.6 What has happened to cerebral blood flow? Is it reversed?

Extra credit Why are manhole covers circular rather than square?

Answers

4.1 The mean arterial pressure at the head would be 50 mm Hg. The hydrostatic pressure at the top of a 200-cm column of arterial blood is 200 mm Hg less than the pressure at the bottom. If the pressure at the bottom (at the level of the heart) is 250 mm Hg, then the pressure at the top is 50 mm Hg.

4.2 The perfusion pressure across the arterial-to-venous pathway is equal to the inlet (cerebral arterial) minus outlet (cerebral venous) pressure. Since the pressure in the cerebral veins is –200 mm Hg, the perfusion pressure is 50 – (–200) = 250 mm Hg.

4.3 The mean arterial pressure at the level of the head is 15 – 200 = –185 mm Hg.

4.4 The venous pressure is also –185 mm Hg, so the arterial-to-venous gradient is 0.

4.5 The cerebral perfusion pressure is 0. It would be a negative number only if you insisted on referencing venous pressure to the level of the heart and referencing arterial pressure to the level of the head. This highlights why it's important to reference all pressures—arterial and venous—to the same level to avoid nonsensical calculations of perfusion pressure.

4.6 No. When properly calculated, cerebral perfusion pressure is 0 and cerebral blood flow is 0.

Extra Credit Only a circular cover will not fall into the manhole if it is removed and turned sideways.

IN THE LOOP—LEFT
VENTRICULAR PRESSURES

WE'VE ALREADY LOOKED AT 2 types of pressure that affect physiology (*atmospheric* and *hydrostatic* pressure). Now let's consider the third: *vascular* pressures that result from mechanical events in the cardiovascular system. As you already know, cardiac output can be defined as the product of heart rate times stroke volume (Figure 5.1). Heart rate is self-explanatory. Stroke volume is determined by 3 factors—preload, afterload, and inotropy—and these determinants are in turn dependent on how the left ventricle handles pressure.

In Figure 5.2, you'll see the standard pressure-volume loop that illustrates the pressure changes that accompany a single cardiac cycle. By the end of this brief chapter, you should be able to draw these things in your sleep. As for the axes, remember that the pressure-volume loop has just exactly those 2 axes, in that order, from left to right. At the corners of the loop are descriptors of the valve events that accompany each pressure transition. "A" is aortic valve and "M" is mitral valve; "O" is opening and "C" is closing. Phase 1 represents ventricular ejection, and the corresponding change on the x-axis represents the stroke volume. Phase 2 is isovolemic (volume not changing) relaxation. Phase 3 is diastolic filling. Phase 4 is isovolemic contraction. With a little bit of thought, you'll see how the corresponding valve events at the corners of the loop define the transitions from one phase to another.

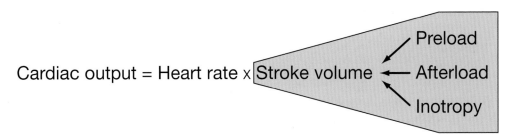

Figure 5.1. Determinants of Cardiac Output.

The E_0 line (pronounced "E-naught") is a little harder to understand. "E" stands for elastance, which is the slope of the pressure/volume relationship (the opposite is compliance, the slope of a volume/pressure relationship). For practical purposes, E_0 defines the boundary (limit) of the ventricle's ability to contract and eject during phase 1. If you don't change inotropy, the E_0 line remains unchanged, and the ventricle can contract only to that line and not beyond it. Figure 5.3 illustrates what happens when inotropy is increased (eg, with epinephrine). The slope of E_0 increases and the ventricle contracts to a lower end-systolic volume during the ejection phase. This means that stroke volume has increased. At the end of isovolumic relaxation, diastolic filling starts at a lower volume as the mitral valve opens. What would happen in a state of decreased inotropy?

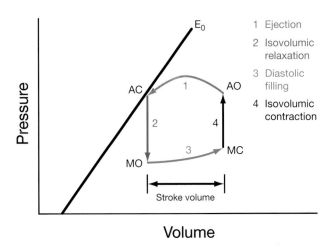

Figure 5.2. Pressure-Volume Loop, Baseline.
A denotes aortic valve; C, closing; E, elastance; M, mitral valve; O, opening.

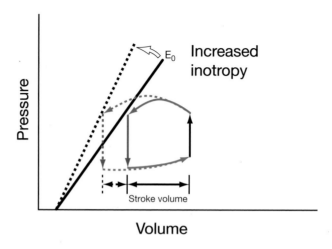

Figure 5.3. Pressure-Volume Loop, Increased Inotropy.
The arrow indicates the direction of change in inotropy.

What happens when preload changes? The original definition of preload was based on experiments with cat papillary muscle that was stretched between 2 points using a strain gauge. In that setting, "preload" meant the degree of stretch before the papillary muscle contracted. For our clinical purposes, "preload" is scaled up from a 1-dimensional stretch to a 3-dimensional volume at the end of diastolic filling. Figure 5.4 shows what happens when preload increases. Diastolic filling extends further to the right before the mitral valve

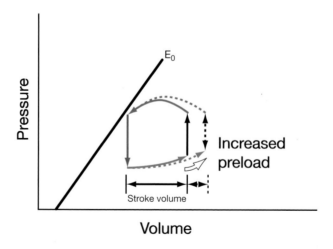

Figure 5.4. Pressure-Volume Loop, Increased Preload.
The arrow indicates the direction of change in preload.

closes and the ventricle contracts—beginning isovolemic contraction. As a result, when the aortic valve opens, ejection occurs at a higher initial volume. If the inotropic state hasn't changed and the E_0 line remains in the same position, ejection proceeds leftward to the same end-systolic volume. This means that stroke volume has increased. What happens when preload decreases?

Finally, Figure 5.5 illustrates what happens with an increase in afterload. In a pressure-volume loop, "afterload" is represented by the pressure at the end of isovolumic contraction—just when the aortic valve opens (because the ventricular pressure is now higher than aortic root pressure). If the inotropic state is unchanged (E_0 slope unchanged), the ejection proceeds to E_0 but at a higher pressure than in the baseline pressure-volume loop. This means that isovolumic relaxation starts at a higher end-systolic volume and stroke volume is decreased. What happens when afterload decreases?

After you master the terminology, these loops not only are straightforward but are easier to construct just by thinking them through, rather than by memorization. In the next chapter, we'll look at the other side of circulation (the venous side) to see what happens with pressures there and how those pressures affect control of cardiac output. This is part of the "standard model" of the cardiovascular system, and you should master it before going on to more interesting applications.

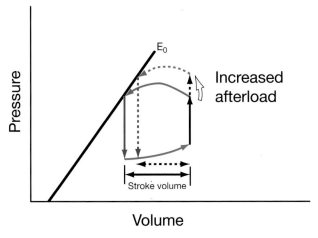

Figure 5.5. Pressure-Volume Loop, Increased Afterload. The arrow indicates the direction of change in preload.

QUESTIONS AND ANSWERS

Questions

5.1 From memory, draw a normal left ventricular pressure-volume loop and label its components. Now superimpose a second loop that demonstrates what happens when preload is decreased.

5.2 Draw another baseline loop and superimpose a second loop illustrating what happens when inotropy and afterload both increase at the same time.

Extra credit Dolphins are mammals that have a sleep requirement (unlike medical students). Nonetheless, they have nowhere to sleep except the open sea. Unlike fish, dolphins are not equipped with swim bladders to maintain neutral buoyancy, and they need to breathe at the surface. How do dolphins manage to satisfy their sleep requirement while remaining afloat?

Answers

5.1

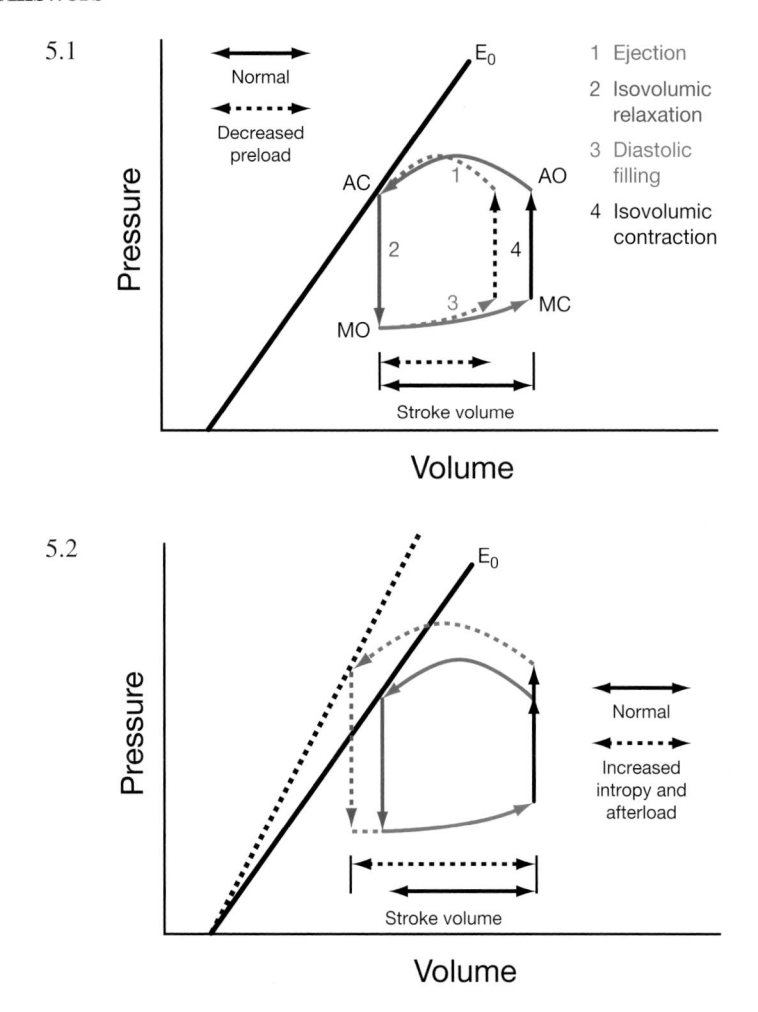

5.2

Extra credit Dolphins are capable of resting 1 cerebral hemisphere at a time, leaving the other hemisphere awake and vigilant.

· 6 ·

WHAT GOES AROUND COMES AROUND—VENOUS RETURN

A TAUTOLOGY IS A circular statement that conveys no new meaning. For example, the phrase "the survival of the fittest" makes very little sense if, by "fittest," we mean "those who survive." The phrase would then be equivalent to saying "the survival of those who survive." By its nature, circulatory physiology is also susceptible to circular reasoning because every part of an interconnected system is affected by, and affects, every other part. If we're not careful, we end up saying things like "venous return equals cardiac output" when, in the steady state, that is true by definition and nothing new is gained.

It's been said that, for an omniscient being, every scientific law is a tautology. Because we're not omniscient, though, we have to pick somewhere in the circulatory system to begin defining all the factors that control cardiac output and just hope that we avoid chasing our tails.

Let's start in the right atrium. If we grant that right atrial pressure (P_{RA}) is the "downstream" pressure for venous return, then it follows that P_{RA} should be inversely related to venous return (and therefore, to cardiac output). What is the "upstream" pressure for venous return? That is a tricky question. The obvious answer would be mean arterial pressure (MAP). After all, we calculate systemic vascular resistance as follows:

$$\text{Systemic vascular resistance} = (\text{MAP} - P_{RA})/\text{CO}$$

where MAP indicates mean arterial pressure; P_{RA}, right atrial pressure; and CO, cardiac output. You may notice that this looks a lot like the hydraulic analogue of Ohm's law of electricity: $V = IR$, where V indicates voltage; I, current; and R, resistance.

Here's where the circular reasoning threatens, however. If we simply apply Ohm's law to the cardiovascular system, we forget that the MAP not only *contributes* to venous return but also is *sustained* by venous return. If venous return fails for any other reason (unrelated to arterial pressure), so too will MAP eventually fail. In that circumstance, we couldn't very well say that the venous return has decreased *because* the gradient between MAP and P_{RA} has decreased when the fall in venous return caused the decreased MAP-P_{RA} gradient in the first place.

You may have anticipated the danger of circular reasoning when I first used the terms "upstream" and "downstream" when describing the circulatory system. That's because every point in a circular system is upstream to one thing and downstream to something else—a bit reminiscent of M.C. Escher's *Waterfall* (Figure 6.1), which gives the illusion of a continuously falling circle of water. Any attempt to pick an arbitrary segment of the circulatory path, with upstream and downstream pressures driving flow, will be susceptible to the danger of circular reasoning.

This isn't just a theoretical objection. It is also borne out by experimental data. Physiologists who have attempted to raise P_{RA} without changing anything else have failed. They have discovered, the hard way, that as P_{RA} increases, venous return and cardiac output decrease to the point at which a decent MAP cannot be sustained and the experiment begins to fall apart. Even if the right atrial function is performed by a mechanical pump, as P_{RA} is raised, the pump begins to fail when it "runs dry" from lack of venous return. There are ways around that practical difficulty (eg, volume loading), but such tactics tend to change other circulatory parameters and just confounds the search for what drives venous return.

When Arthur Guyton first performed his venous return curve experiments in the 1950s, he encountered the same phenomenon. To define the relationship between P_{RA} and venous return, he increased P_{RA} (the independent variable) and measured venous return

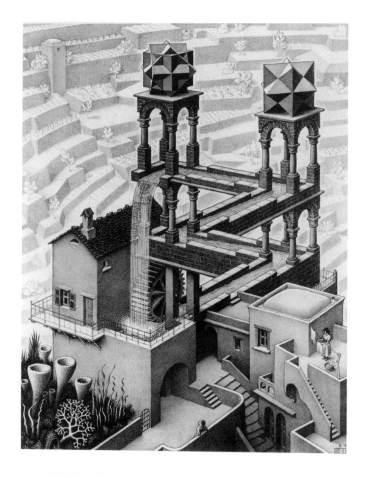

Figure 6.1. Waterfall.

(From M.C. Escher's "Waterfall." ©2010 The M.C. Escher Company-Holland. All rights reserved. www.mcescher.com. Used with permission.)

(the dependent variable). If MAP was the relevant upstream pressure for venous return, then he should have been able to increase P_{RA} until it was the same as MAP before the gradient was abolished and venous return decreased to zero. As you can now predict, that didn't happen. What did happen was this: as P_{RA} rose, venous return fell, the right atrial bypass pump began to run dry and fail, and MAP fell. This occurred when P_{RA} was only about 15 mm Hg—in other words, when P_{RA} approached what physiologists call *mean systemic pressure* (P_{ms}), the pressure that every part of the cardiovascular system equilibrates to during cardiac arrest. It was on this basis that P_{ms} was designated as the "upstream pressure" for venous return.

Taking that result and applying Ohm's law again to the cardiovascular system, venous return can be calculated as follows:

$$\textbf{Venous return} = (P_{ms} - P_{RA})/R_v$$

where P_{ms} indicates mean systemic pressure; P_{RA}, right atrial pressure; and R_v, resistance to venous return. This relationship allowed Guyton to construct the venous return curve, relating P_{RA} to venous return (Figure 6.2).

When P_{RA} is as high as P_{ms}, there is no gradient for venous return and no flow occurs. As P_{RA} decreases, venous return increases. This "curve" would be a simple straight line with a negative slope (proportional to R_v), except that something funny happens when the P_{RA} is subatmospheric (ie, when a catheter is put in the right atrium and siphoned to a lower level, or when suction is applied to the right atrium [as is done in some patients with a "vacuum-assist device" in the pump]). At subatmospheric pressures, the thoracic veins tend to collapse (see the chapter on the Starling resistor [Chapter 15]—this

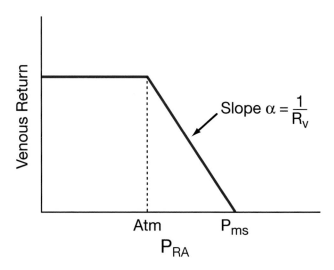

Figure 6.2. Venous Return Curve.

Atm denotes atmospheric; P_{ms}, mean systemic pressure; P_{RA}, right atrial pressure; R_v, resistance to venous return.

is an example of one). Once the veins begin to collapse, there is no longer an incremental increase in venous return as P_{RA} decreases, and the venous return curve begins to plateau.

If you accept Guyton's premise that we can talk about a "gradient for venous return" without getting into circular reasoning, then this type of venous return curve and the equation for venous return are very useful ways to define the parameters. As you'll see in the next chapter, Guyton took this approach one step further by superimposing the venous return curve on a cardiac function curve that relates P_{RA} to cardiac output. This is a very clever way of defending what would seem to be an arbitrary segmentation of the circulatory system, and it avoids using circular logic when defining the control of venous return.

QUESTIONS AND ANSWERS

Questions

6.1 Draw a normal venous return curve and label its components.

6.2 Why is venous return zero when right atrial pressure is the same as mean systemic pressure?

Extra credit The old Russian postal system was notoriously corrupt. Anything other than a mailed letter was opened and stolen, regardless of value. Locked packages or boxes were left alone, however, because they were too much trouble to pry open and the other pickings were so good. Boris lived in Moscow and Natasha lived in St. Petersburg. Neither could leave their home city, but Boris wanted to send a gem to Natasha without it being stolen. He had a lock box with a hasp that could accommodate padlocks. Boris called Natasha and they devised a scheme to get the jewel to her safely. They had access only to key locks (no combination locks), but a key could not be sent through the mail in an envelope because it would be stolen, even if the key had no value to the thief. How did Boris get the gem to Natasha? (Adapted from Flannery S, Flannery D. In code: a mathematical journey. New York: Workman Publishing Company; 2001. p. 16–17. Used with permission.)

Answers

6.1

6.2 Because the pressure gradient for venous return is the difference between mean systemic pressure (P_{ms}) and right atrial pressure (P_{RA}), if P_{RA} equals P_{ms}, no gradient for venous return exists and no venous return will occur.

Extra credit Boris put the gem in the lock box, attached a lock to the hasp, and mailed the box to Natasha. On receipt, Natasha placed her own lock on the same hasp and mailed the box back to Boris, with both locks in place. Boris removed his lock and returned the box to Natasha, who removed her lock, opened the box, and retrieved the gem.

· 7 ·

PUSHMI-PULLYU AND
THE RIGHT ATRIUM

HERE'S A SIMPLE QUESTION with a not-so-simple answer—what does right atrial pressure (P_{RA}) do to cardiac output (CO)? On the one hand, we've been taught that P_{RA} represents preload for the right ventricle. That is, the higher the P_{RA}, the greater the right ventricular output (and, therefore, CO). This is simply an application of Starling's law to the right side of the heart. On the other hand, we've been taught that P_{RA} represents the downstream impedance to venous return (VR) from the periphery. That is, the higher the P_{RA}, the lower the VR, and therefore, the *lower* the CO. So, which is it? Is a higher P_{RA} good or bad for CO?

In the 1950s, physiologist Arthur Guyton attempted to solve this apparently circular problem by breaking the circle and analyzing the "cut" ends. In essence, Guyton treated the P_{RA} as Dr Dolittle's mythical "pushmi-pullyu," which had 2 heads facing in opposite directions (Figure 7.1). In his analysis, the P_{RA} *simultaneously* served as the right ventricular preload (a good thing) and impedance to VR (a bad thing). How can that be done? One way is to draw 2 separate curves on the same graph—one represents CO as a function of P_{RA} (a classic Starling curve for the right side of the heart), and the other represents VR as a function of P_{RA} (Figure 7.2).

Because P_{RA} is assumed to be the independent variable for both curves (ie, the cause of CO and the cause of VR), the 2 graphs may

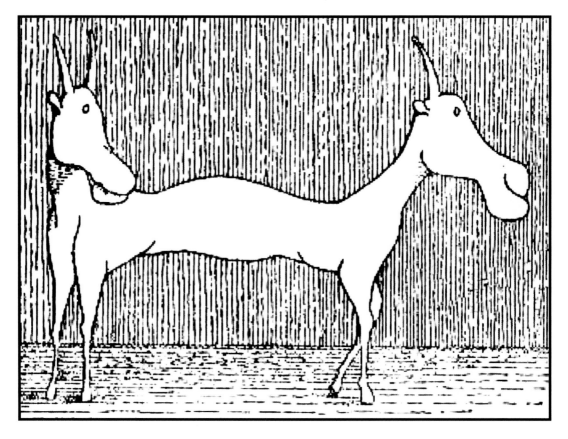

Figure 7.1. Pushmi-pullyu, the mythical animal from Hugh Lofting's *The Story of Doctor Dolittle*. (Adapted from Lofting H. The Story of Doctor Dolittle. New York: Frederick A. Stokes Company; 1920.)

be superimposed, with P_{RA} on the x-axis (Figure 7.3). The y-axis may be designated as flow because VR and CO both are measured in liters of blood per minute.

Guyton reasoned that the intersection of the 2 curves represented the one unique point at which everything settled into a peaceful compromise of forces. That special point defined *both* CO and VR because, in the steady state, they are equal by definition. In fact, the constraint that CO equals VR was essential to this approach because it served as the mathematical link between the 2 separate curves. In other words, if you didn't know anything else about the relationship between P_{RA} and the cardiac function curve ahead of that point or between P_{RA} and the VR curve behind that point, you would at least know that the 2 functions intersected at 1 unique blood flow rate.

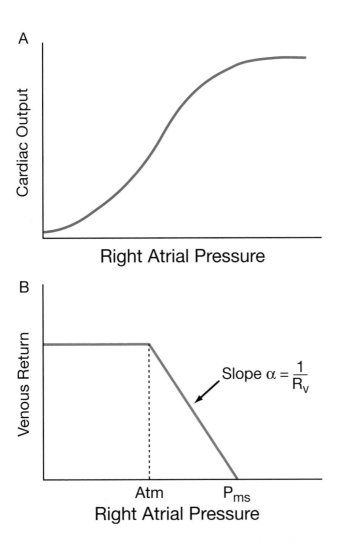

Figure 7.2.   A, Cardiac Output Curve (Starling's Law of the Heart). B, Venous Return Curve. Atm denotes atmospheric; P_{ms}, mean systemic pressure; R_v, resistance to venous return.

You have already seen in Chapter 6 (What Goes Around Comes Around—Venous Return) and will see again in Chapter 9 (Down But Not Out—Circulatory Arrest Pressures) what defines the VR curve. Now, let's look at the intersection of the VR and cardiac function curves when they're plotted together (Figure 7.3). You'll notice that the CO curve (Starling curve) demonstrates that output increases as a function of increasing P_{RA}—that is, P_{RA} functions as preload. In contrast, P_{RA} is inversely related to the VR for the sloping portion of the VR curve. The point of intersection between

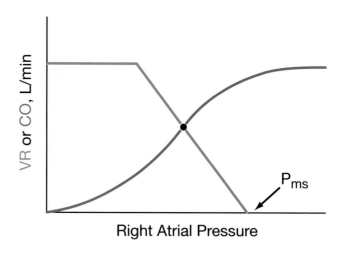

Figure 7.3.   Relationship Between VR and CO.

CO denotes cardiac output; P_{ms}, mean systemic pressure; VR, venous return.

the 2 curves defines a unique blood flow rate, which is both CO and VR at the same time.

One nice mathematical feature of Guyton's analysis is that it can predict changes in overall CO in response to an isolated change in any of the variables that define VR. For example, if a change in blood volume affects VR, the VR curve shifts and the VR and

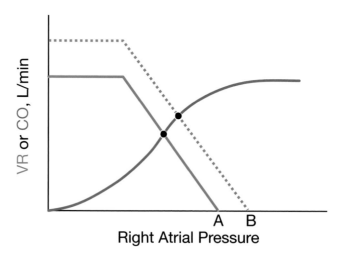

Figure 7.4.   Volume Loading.

Note that mean systemic pressure increases from A to B with volume loading. CO denotes cardiac output; VR, venous return.

CO curves intersect at a new point (Figure 7.4). If you're paying attention, you might notice that this new intersection point not only defines a new CO (y-axis value of the intersection point), it also defines a new P_{RA} (x-axis value of the new intersection point).

Have another look at Figure 7.4. Remember from our previous discussion that the VR curve intersects the x-axis at the mean systemic pressure (P_{ms}). P_{ms} is simply the ratio of stressed blood volume to vascular compliance; therefore, when we perform volume loading on a patient, the P_{ms} increases (from A to B on the graph). This shifts the VR curve to the right without affecting the CO curve. By Guyton's analysis, we can look at the new intersection point between the VR and CO curves and predict that CO will be slightly higher. We can also predict the new P_{RA} by looking at the horizontal shift of the intersection point.

This type of analysis is so useful because it answers an otherwise very difficult question. We know that a central venous pressure catheter measures pressure very close to the right atrium. We also know, from experience, that volume loading results in a rise in central venous pressure. However, we have been taught that a healthy heart accommodates an increased load by pumping out more blood (Starling's law of the heart again); that, in turn, should lower central venous pressure back toward where it started. Guyton's

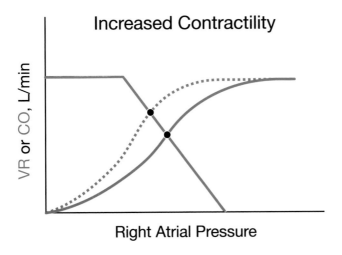

Figure 7.5. Increased Contractility.

CO denotes cardiac output; VR, venous return.

superimposition of the VR and CO curves allows us to predict, both qualitatively and quantitatively, where the P_{RA} will be after volume loading.

The same analysis works for other changes in VR or cardiac function parameters. For example, if you were wondering what happens when inotropy (contractility) increases, just shift the cardiac function curve to the left (dotted line) and leave the VR curve alone (Figure 7.5). The new intersection point predicts a higher CO and VR and also predicts lower P_{RA}. That's exactly what happens in real life.

What you've just learned is the standard textbook model for VR. You should always know the dogma before you challenge it—besides, it's the dogma that you'll be tested on. The next chapter will present you with an interesting logical challenge to Guyton's foundational work.

QUESTIONS AND ANSWERS

Questions

7.1 Draw a normal venous return curve and superimpose a normal cardiac function curve. On the same graph, demonstrate what happens with simultaneous increased inotropy and volume loading.

7.2 What does a venous return–cardiac function curve tell you that a pressure-volume loop does not?

Extra credit You start hiking from the bottom of Mt. Rainier at 6:00 AM and reach the summit at 6:00 PM. After spending the night on the summit, you begin hiking down at 6:00 AM the next day, following the same route, and reach the bottom at 6:00 PM. Regardless of how often you took breaks or varied your speed on the ascent and descent, explain why there must be 1 point on the trail where you were present at exactly the same time of day on both trips.

Answers

7.1

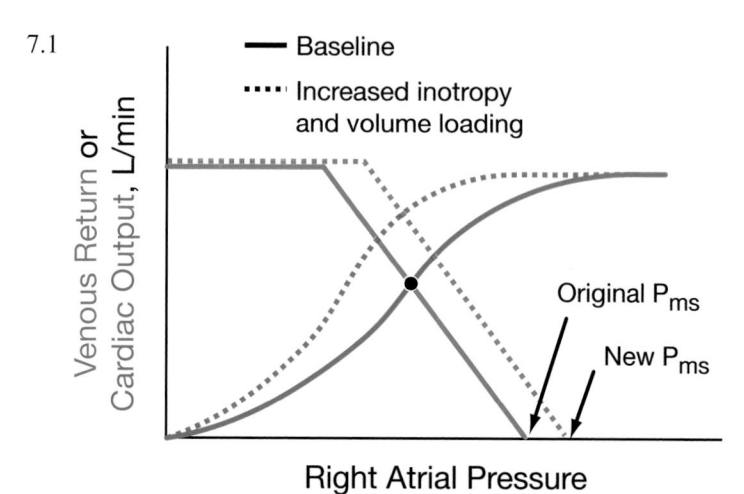

7.2 The left ventricular pressure-volume curve predicts the effects of inotropy, preload, and afterload on stroke volume. In contrast, a venous return–cardiac function curve predicts the reciprocal interactions between the arterial and venous sides of the systemic circulation. It also predicts the right atrial pressure resulting from these interactions.

Extra credit You can depict the 2 trips as functions on the same graph, with time on the x-axis and altitude on the y-axis. Both functions begin at 6:00 AM and end at 6:00 PM. The ascent begins at base elevation and ends at summit elevation. The descent begins at summit elevation and ends at base elevation. No matter the profile of each function, they will cross at some point. At that intersection, you were at the same place at the same time on both trips.

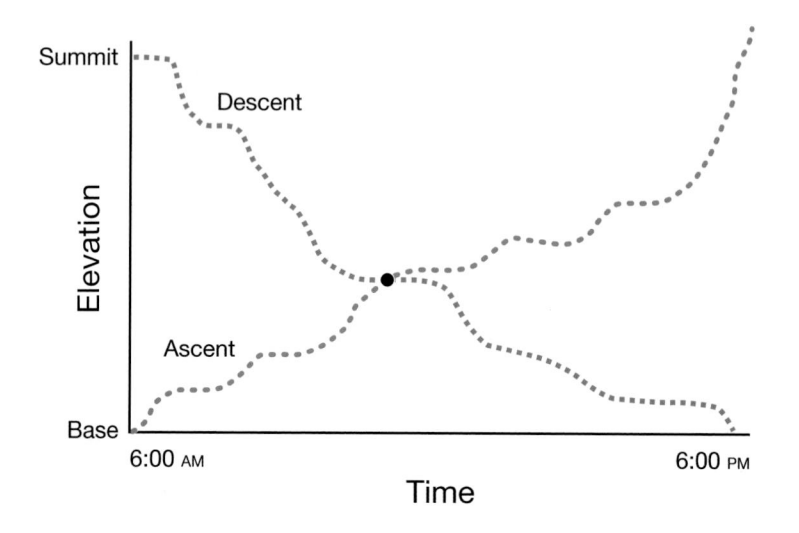

· 8 ·

PRESSURE AND FLOW—
CHICKENS AND EGGS

MOST OF US AREN'T statisticians. Socially, that's probably a good thing. Occasionally, though, it gets us into trouble. For example, we tend to assume that when 2 things are associated with each other, one must be *causing* the other. Nothing could be further from the truth, though. Take the example of the steamboat in Figure 8.1. A steam engine powers the paddle wheel, and the turning action of the paddle wheel propels the boat forward. As the wheel churns through the water, it digs a temporary "trough" and displaces water into a small raised wake behind the wheel. As a result, a hydrostatic pressure gradient develops between the peak of the wake and the trough below it. We could estimate that pressure gradient very easily by measuring the vertical height between peak and trough ($P_1 - P_2$) and multiplying that height by the density of water and the acceleration due to gravity (pressure gradient = ρgh).

In fact, we could go one step further and measure the relationship between the paddle wheel flow rate and the hydrostatic pressure gradient. Suppose that we did that and found that they were related by a constant: $K (P_1 - P_2)$ = paddle wheel flow rate. We could even construct a graph (Figure 8.2) and proclaim a new physical law, the "Law of Paddle Wheels."

Because we're used to seeing the independent variable ("cause") plotted on the x-axis and the dependent variable ("effect") on the

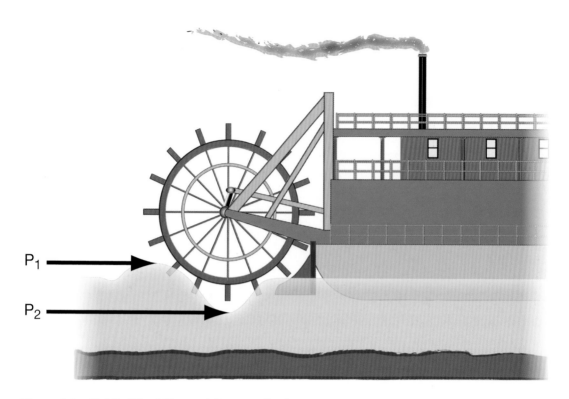

Figure 8.1. Paddle Wheel Flow and Pressure Gradient.

Does the gradient cause the flow, or does the flow cause the gradient?

y-axis, this equation and graph suggest that the pressure gradient *causes* the paddle wheel flow rate. That, of course, is nonsense. This type of specious thinking is intended to warn you away from assuming that relationships necessarily imply causality.

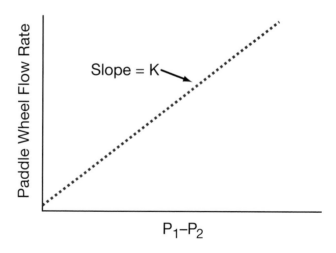

Figure 8.2. The "Law" of Paddle Wheels.

It was just this sort of logical skepticism about cause and effect that motivated physiologist Matthew Levy to question the conventional wisdom surrounding Arthur Guyton's venous return curves and their accompanying equation:

$$\textbf{Venous return} = (\textbf{P}_{ms} - \textbf{P}_{RA})/\textbf{R}_v$$

where P_{ms} indicates mean systemic pressure; P_{RA}, right atrial pressure; and R_v, resistance to venous return.

Simply put, Levy questioned the assignment of dependent and independent variables in the standard venous return analysis that you previously learned. To Levy, it didn't necessarily follow that a tight mathematical relationship between venous return, the pressure gradient, and the calculated resistance for venous return meant that the gradient for venous return *caused* venous return. In fact, in a very simple experiment, he demonstrated that flow was more likely the cause (not the effect) of pressure gradients within the cardiovascular system.

Levy placed an anesthetized dog on cardiopulmonary bypass and measured central venous and arterial pressures while directly controlling blood flow rate with the bypass pump. Just as Starling had demonstrated a century before, when flow was stopped (pump shut off), arterial and venous pressures converged to mean systemic pressure. As the pump flow rate was turned up, arterial pressures rose and central venous pressures fell in direct proportion to the flow rate (Figure 8.3). In this case, Levy reasoned, it was pretty hard to argue that flow was anything other than the *cause* and pressure gradients anything other than the *effect*.

As you might imagine, this interpretation caused a bit of a debate between Levy and Guyton. The essence of that discussion was nicely summarized in an appendix to the article (see Figure 8.3 legend for the reference), and it makes worthwhile reading for anyone interested in physiology.

We certainly won't settle their debate here, but it is worth noting that Levy may have thermodynamics on his side. As you've learned already, pressure is not the same thing as energy, and pressure by itself cannot perform work or generate flow. However,

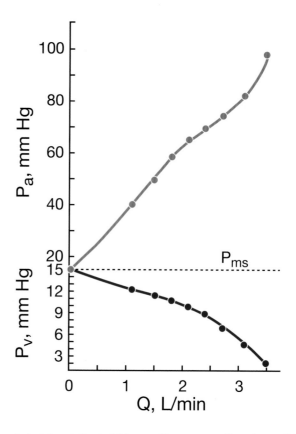

Figure 8.3. Arterial and Central Venous Pressures as Functions of Systemic Blood Flow.

P_a denotes arterial pressure; P_{ms}, mean systemic pressure; P_v, venous pressure; Q, systemic blood flow. Note that the scales for P_a and P_v are not the same. (Adapted from Levy MN. The cardiac and vascular factors that determine systemic blood flow. Circ Res. 1979 Jun;44[6]:739-47. Used with permission.)

flow generated by pressure-volume work (either by the heart or a mechanical pump) certainly can create pressure gradients. In this sort of chicken (flow) or egg (pressure) question (Figure 8.4), if the only energy-containing term is flow, then I'll say that the chicken came first.

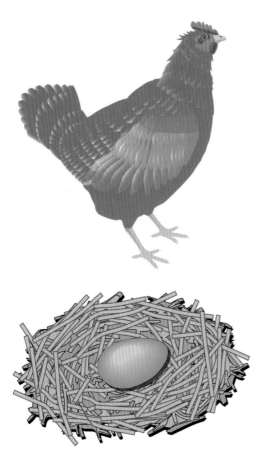

Figure 8.4.   Chicken and Egg.

QUESTIONS AND ANSWERS

Questions

8.1 Think of a circumstance in which you have 2 variables with a very tight, reproducible, and quantitative relationship but no direct cause-and-effect relationship.

8.2 What would a statistical test of correlation between ice cream sales and violent crime show?

8.3 What lesson can you derive from this exercise with regard to the use (or misuse) of graphs and statistical tests of correlation?

Extra credit A rope is placed around the circumference of the Earth at the equator. Assume that the surface of the Earth is completely smooth and that it is a perfect sphere. Now imagine the rope is lengthened by 1 m. When the lengthened rope is pulled uniformly away from the Earth's surface, parallel to the equator, a gap will form between the rope and the planet surface. How big is the gap? Does the size of the gap depend on the radius of the Earth? (Adapted from Flannery S, Flannery D. In code: a mathematical journey. New York: Workman Publishing Company; 2001. p. 21–22. Used with permission.)

Answers

8.1 It is important to distinguish between correlation and causality. Consider the example of the relationship between ice cream sales and violent crime. Each correlates with warm weather and, therefore, with one another. This does not mean, however, that one causes the other.

8.2 A statistical test would likely show a significant correlation, but again, this does not mean that one causes the other.

8.3 The lesson is the same for physiology as for other aspects of life. In this chapter, we saw that pressure gradients correlate with flow. That does not mean, however, that pressure gradients cause flow. One could argue that flow is the result of a gradient in total fluid energy (which is not always reflected in a gradient of pressure) and that pressure gradients are the result of flow through a resistance. The experiment by Matthew Levy illustrated just that point. By convention, we plot the independent variable ("cause") on the x-axis and the dependent variable ("effect") on the y-axis. In the graph from Levy's simple experiment, he correctly placed blood flow on the x-axis and pressure gradients on the y-axis.

Extra credit The resulting gap is approximately 0.16 m wide, and the size of the gap does NOT depend on the radius of the Earth. If 1 meter was added to a rope around a beach ball and pulled uniformly away from the surface, the resulting gap would still be 0.16 m. As counterintuitive as this solution seems, it is true. The proof is a matter of simple algebra—the initial radius (or circumference) of the sphere cancels out and therefore has no effect on the solution.

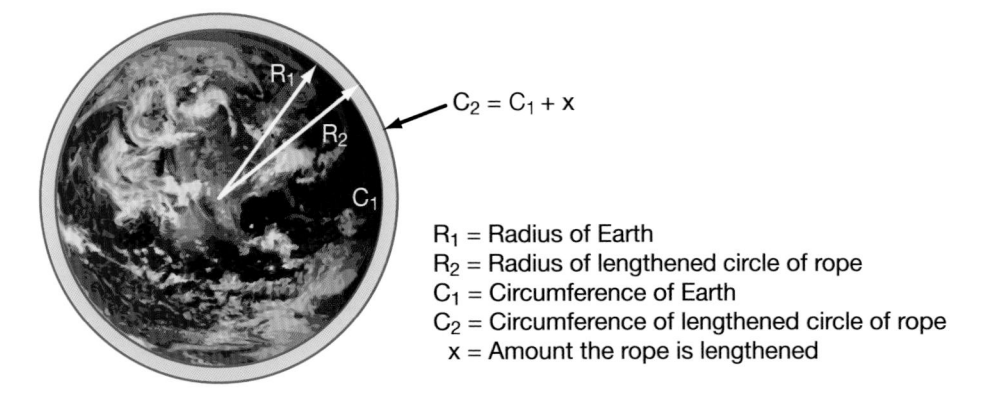

$C_2 = C_1 + x$

R_1 = Radius of Earth
R_2 = Radius of lengthened circle of rope
C_1 = Circumference of Earth
C_2 = Circumference of lengthened circle of rope
x = Amount the rope is lengthened

$$R_1 = C_1/2\pi \qquad R_2 = (C_1+x)/2\pi$$

$$R_2-R_1 = (C_1+x)/2\pi - C_1/2\pi = x/2\pi$$

For an initial lengthening of 1 m: $1/2\pi \approx 0.16$ m

This difference is independent of the initial circumference!

DOWN BUT NOT OUT—CIRCULATORY ARREST PRESSURES

THE CEREBRAL ANGIOGRAM IN Figure 9.1 shows a 5-cm aneurysm of the internal carotid artery. You won't find many neurosurgeons willing to repair an aneurysm this big, but if you do, they will most likely insist that the surgery take place with the patient under deep hypothermic circulatory arrest. During the brief (about 30-minute) arrest phase, very little can go wrong because most of the patient's physiologic functions are already absent. In addition to the issues of deep hypothermia (18°C), these cases also present some fascinating aspects of circulatory physiology because we are intentionally bringing the whole cardiovascular system to a standstill.

Let's think through that for a moment. Suppose that your heart has just stopped. What would happen to your blood pressure? At least 2 things would happen that you might not predict (and I hope you won't discover them anytime soon). First, the various blood pressures in the different parts of your circulatory system would converge to the same value. That includes arterial, capillary, venous, pulmonary, left atrial, and left ventricular pressures—you name it, they're all going to be the same. Why is that? By Pascal's principle, a change in pressure in a fluid is equally distributed throughout the fluid at the same hydrostatic level. Remember that the pumping heart supplies fluid energy and flow, and flow creates pressure gradients in the cardiovascular system. If the heart stops, the energy source to maintain

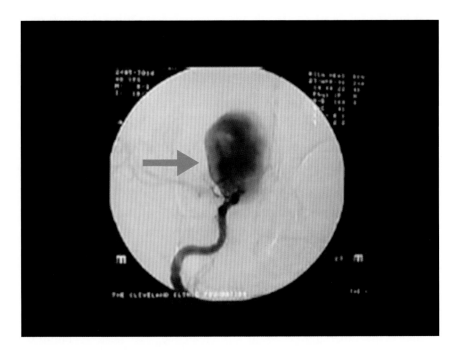

Figure 9.1. Cerebral Angiogram Shows a Large Aneurysm.

pressure gradients is absent, so all pressures will converge to the same value. What about the valves? Can valves maintain pressure gradients during cardiac arrest? The answer is "no." Valves prevent only backward flow, not forward flow, and forward flow is sufficient to allow pressure equilibration throughout the circulatory system.

Second, you might be surprised to find that your blood pressure is not zero. That's not just because of vertical (hydrostatic) gradients within the body. Because the blood volume is considerably greater than the passive circulatory system volume, the blood vessels are slightly stretched and maintain a non-zero pressure even after the heart stops. Imagine that you are filling a large balloon with water and keeping track of the balloon volume and the pressure inside the balloon. You would have to add a certain amount of water (a sort of "priming volume") before the walls of the balloon began to stretch and generate pressure.

The passive or "unstretched" circulatory volume (about 2 L in an adult) is termed *unstressed volume* (V_0). It's easy to remember that term because the unstressed volume is the same thing as the unstretched volume. Only the blood volume in excess of the unstressed volume of the circulatory system contributes to pressure. This, of course, is termed the *stressed blood volume*, and it is calculated as follows: $V - V_0$, where V indicates total blood volume and V_0, unstressed volume.

When we take care of trauma patients, we worry a lot about stressed blood volume because that is the only thing keeping them alive. For reasons that will become apparent as you learn more about circulatory physiology, if the blood volume is at or below the unstressed volume, the heart cannot generate a physiologically meaningful blood pressure, regardless of how hard or fast it contracts. For now, I will just tell you that if the total blood volume is below V_0, there is not enough blood returning from the periphery to the heart, and the heart therefore cannot generate pressure or flow.

We know changes in total blood volume can occur with hemorrhage, transfusion, intravenous fluid administration, renal function, and many other things. What can change V_0? At least 2 conditions come to mind. One is pathologic vasodilation—some time after a patient dies, the blood vessels dilate and V_0 will *increase* to the point where the total blood volume is producing little or no pressure. The second cause is a positional change. When we place a patient in a head-down (Trendelenberg) position, we have effectively removed that portion of blood volume in the legs from V_0 (V_0 will *decrease*).

To determine the actual non-zero pressure during cardiac arrest, we only have to divide the stressed blood volume by vascular compliance. Remember that compliance is the ratio of volume to pressure ($\Delta V/\Delta P$ or dV/dP), so volume divided by compliance yields pressure. The non-zero arrest pressure is termed *mean systemic pressure* (P_{ms}). This should not be confused with *systolic pressure*—systemic and systolic have nothing to do with each other. The formula for calculating P_{ms} is as follows (remember this because we'll use it later): $P_{ms} = (V - V_0)/C_v$, where P_{ms} indicates mean systemic pressure; V, total blood volume; V_0, unstressed volume; and C_v, vascular compliance. This isn't rocket science, is it? Most of the important equations and relationships in physiology are as simple as this one.

There are very few clinical situations in which we can unmask a normal P_{ms}. I don't include cardiac arrests that occur in the context of trauma because they are usually accompanied by significant changes in volume and vascular compliance. One situation that I can think of is a planned circulatory arrest performed under deep hypothermia, like the one depicted in Figure 9.2. The panels show arterial pressure, pulmonary arterial pressure, peripheral venous pressure, and central venous pressure before bypass is initiated, on bypass during cooling, just as the bypass pump is shut off, and during arrest. The venous drainage line to the venous reservoir was clamped simultaneously with discontinuation of bypass so that the patient's blood volume remained unchanged during the arrest phase.

Notice that the arrested circulation does not go to zero pressure (just as you've been taught). During the arrest phase, the patient's blood volume and vascular tone are relatively preserved, and all pressures converge to a P_{ms} of about 10 to 15 mm Hg (Figure 9.2D). That

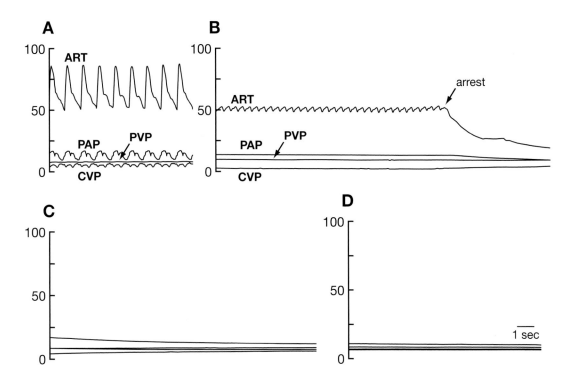

Figure 9.2. Hemodynamic Variables During Controlled Circulatory Arrest.

A, Before cardiopulmonary bypass. B, Immediately before and during circulatory arrest. C and D, Continuation of panel B. ART denotes arterial blood pressure; CVP, central venous pressure; PAP, pulmonary artery blood pressure; PVP, peripheral venous pressure. (Adapted from Munis JR, Bhatia S, Lozada LJ. Peripheral venous pressure as a hemodynamic variable in neurosurgical patients. Anesth Analg. 2001;92:172-9. Used with permission.)

is precisely what physiologist Arthur Guyton predicted on the basis of animal experiments performed in the 1950s. In one of Guyton's classic papers, he commented that we would probably never be able to determine P_{ms} in humans. He couldn't have known in 1957 that we would someday be able to do the type of anesthetic procedure that allows direct measurement of P_{ms}.

If you observed this patient during the hypothermic arrest phase, you might notice that there is no physiologic evidence of life. Each "vital sign" is absent. Nevertheless, as long as the arrest phase is brief, we can retrieve the patient from this suspended animation state.

QUESTIONS AND ANSWERS

Questions

9.1 What are 3 ways of increasing mean systemic pressure?

9.2 Is there one place in each systemic circulation loop where the blood pressure doesn't change, even if the heart stops? If so, approximately where anatomically do you think that point might be?

Extra credit Do surgical patients in Denver bleed more than their counterparts in New York City because of lower atmospheric pressure surrounding their open capillaries? Why or why not?

Answers

9.1 1) Increase total blood volume. 2) Decrease vascular compliance. 3) Decrease unstressed blood volume.

9.2 Yes. Because the pressure in the aorta is higher than the circulatory arrest pressure (ie, the mean systemic pressure) and the pressure in the right atrium is lower than circulatory arrest pressure, it is mathematically necessary that one point between the aorta and the right atrium has a pressure that is identical to circulatory arrest pressure. This occurs in the small peripheral veins.

Extra credit No. Because blood vessels are compliant and the soft tissues between vessels and the surface of the body are also compliant, the pressure of the atmosphere at the surface of the body is added to the total vascular pressure. By Pascal's principle, the pressure from the atmosphere, which opposes blood leakage from a vessel into the air, is distributed equally throughout the vascular system. As a result, any change in atmospheric pressure will affect equally the pressure inside a leaking capillary and the air pressure outside of the same capillary, and the 2 pressures cancel each other out.

STARLING'S RIDDLE OF
THE BROKEN HEART

A LITTLE MORE THAN a hundred years ago, the physiologist
Ernest Starling told a story and asked a riddle. His audience, shel-
tered from a London winter inside the halls of the Royal College of
Surgeons, came to hear about heart failure (Figure 10.1).

"So what was there to hear?" you might ask a comfortable century later. "After all, the heart is a pump, and when it fails for any
reason, the blood doesn't circulate as it should, various parts of
the body swell with congestion, and the story ends unhappily. That
hardly sounds like something to trudge through a London February
to hear. Maybe the food was good?"

When Ernest Starling lectured, however, there was usually something remarkable to hear. The experiment that Starling highlighted
was very simple. He placed a catheter into the pericardium of an
anesthetized dog and slowly infused oil into it. This produced an
incremental cardiac tamponade, ie, a form of acute heart failure.
During the process, Starling recorded pressures in the femoral artery,
portal vein, and vena cava. I've replotted his data in Figure 10.2.

Something striking occurred when the tamponade began to have
an effect (about 70 mL infused). The arterial pressure began to fall,
of course, but the venous pressures began to rise. In other words,
heart failure didn't just decrease one type of pressure, it simultaneously increased another type of pressure. In fact, by the end of

𝕿𝖍𝖊 𝕬𝖗𝖗𝖎𝖘 𝖆𝖓𝖉 𝕲𝖆𝖑𝖊 𝕷𝖊𝖈𝖙𝖚𝖗𝖊𝖘

ON

SOME POINTS IN THE PATHOLOGY OF HEART DISEASE

Delivered at the Royal College of Surgeons of England on Feb. 22nd, 24th, and 26th, 1897,
By ERNEST H. STARLING, M.D.,
M.R.C.P. Lond.,
JOINT LECTURES ON PHYSIOLOGY AT GUY'S HOSPITAL

LECTURE II.
Delivered on Feb. 24th.
THE EFFECTS OF HEART FAILURE ON THE CIRCULATION.

Figure 10.1. Starling Lecture.

(Adapted from Starling EH. Some points in the pathology of heart disease [lecture]. Lancet. 1897 Mar 6;149[3836]:652-5.)

the experiment, all pressures had converged to the same value. If you remember Chapter 9 (Down But Not Out—Circulatory Arrest Pressures), you know that they converged to the mean systemic pressure (P_{ms}), which is simply the ratio of stressed blood volume to vascular compliance. And, as it was with Guyton's experiments a half century later, the P_{ms} in Starling's experiment was about 15 mm Hg.

Before we get to Starling's riddle, let's review what we have so far because, while it is not too surprising, neither is it obvious. The heart, like any pump, doesn't just raise fluid pressure on one side, it simultaneously lowers fluid pressure on the opposite side. Think of the electrical analogy to the pump: the battery. Batteries have a similar property—they don't just raise voltage on one side, they lower voltage on the other side at the same time.

If you don't believe that the heart lowers venous pressure as it raises arterial pressure, consider the ingenious experiment performed by Dr E.H. Sonnenblick, who confirmed that the heart can

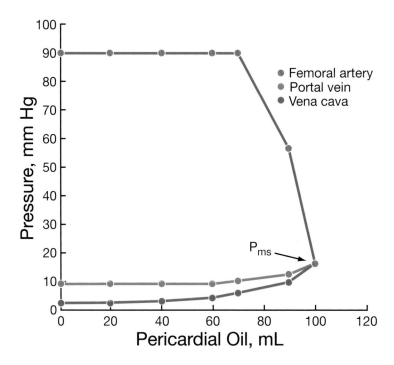

Figure 10.2. Effect of Tamponade on Arterial and Venous Pressures.

P_{ms} denotes mean systemic pressure. (Data from Starling EH. Some points in the pathology of heart disease [lecture]. Lancet. 1897 Mar 6;149[3836]:652-5.)

function as a suction pump. If a freshly excised, still-beating ventricle is placed in a beaker of saline, it does something peculiar—it repeatedly propels itself through the liquid with each beat, just like a squid. If the ventricle were not "sucking" liquid into its chamber with each diastole (relaxation), it would do that trick only once before lying flaccid and mostly empty, unable to fill and stretch itself again for another squirt. The heart has a peculiar architecture that prefers a slightly filled resting state. Any smaller volume actually requires active contraction—it passively springs open during a part of diastole, suctioning blood into itself. Thus, we can go a bit further than just stating that a pump can lower pressure on one side as it raises pressure on the other; for the heart, it *must* lower pressure on the intake side during part of its pumping cycle.

Let's go back to Starling. He was one of the first physiologists to describe P_{ms}, the non-zero cardiac arrest pressure. But he noticed something more. P_{ms}, which was about 15 mm Hg, was *less* than the pressure of most capillaries. Of course, there is a broad range of capillary pressures in the body, but it's fair to say that 25 mm Hg is a reasonable estimate.

Now have a look at Figure 10.3, which plots blood pressure as a function of distance through the systemic circulation, from the aorta to the right atrium (this graph neglects systolic pressure fluctuations). The dotted horizontal line is cardiac arrest pressure (P_{ms}). As the heart fails, the left-hand side of the pressure decay curve decreases to converge with the dotted line, and the right-hand part of the pressure decay curve increases to converge with the same line. At complete cardiac arrest, all pressures will coincide exactly with the P_{ms} line at 15 mm Hg. Notice where the capillary pressure is located on this graph—it is *above* the P_{ms}. In other words, heart failure should cause the average capillary pressure to decrease, not increase.

So, here is Starling's riddle: why does heart failure cause capillary edema? We understand that the pressure in large veins (right-hand side of the pressure decay curve) will rise with heart failure, but capillary pressure is on the left side of the intersection of the curve and the P_{ms} line. As such, capillary pressure should decrease

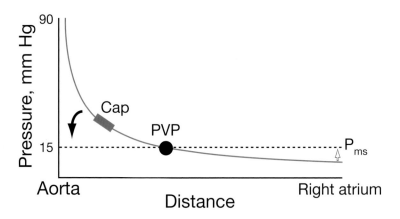

Figure 10.3. Blood Pressure Decay Curve.

The plot shows blood pressure as a function of distance from the aorta to the right atrium. During heart failure, the left side of the pressure decay curve decreases to converge with P_{ms} (black arrow), whereas the right side of the curve increases to converge with P_{ms} (white arrow). Cap denotes capillary pressure; P_{ms}, mean systemic pressure; PVP, peripheral venous pressure. (Adapted from Munis JR, Bhatia S, Lozada LJ. Peripheral venous pressure as a hemodynamic variable in neurosurgical patients. Anesth Analg. 2001 Jan;92[1]:172-9. Used with permission.)

(not increase) with heart failure, and the tendency toward edema similarly should decrease.

When I teach this hundred-year-old lesson to students and residents, I point out that acute, right-sided heart failure doesn't cause peripheral edema, even though we know that patients with *chronic* (congestive) heart failure get peripheral edema, just like the textbooks say they should. In response to this paradox, students usually suggest that there isn't enough time for edema formation in the acute setting. They are right—but for the wrong reason. It isn't that edema takes very long (anesthesiologists know better, at least when it comes to pulmonary edema, but that's a different story). Instead, the answer is that chronic heart failure is accompanied by fluid retention and an increase in blood volume. The greater volume in turn increases P_{ms}—on the graph in Figure 10.3, it raises the dotted line above capillary pressure, and with greater capillary pressure, edema occurs.

This teaches us that a failing heart can do only 2 things to the pressure in any given systemic blood vessel. If the vessel pressure plots to the left of the intersection between the decay curve and the P_{ms} line (eg, the capillaries), heart failure will *decrease* the vessel pressure. If the vessel pressure plots to the right of the intersection point (eg, the portal vein or vena cava in Starling's experiment), heart failure will *increase* the vessel pressure, although never higher than P_{ms}. Neither situation will cause edema formation. Edema will occur only when right-sided heart failure is accompanied by an increased P_{ms} from volume retention.

In addition to making these simple but elegant observations, Ernest Starling described the intravascular forces responsible for edema formation. Accordingly, they are known as "Starling Forces":

$$Q = K\,[(P_c - P_i) - \sigma(\pi_c - \pi_i)]$$

where Q denotes edema rate; K, a filtration coefficient; P_c, pressure within the capillary; P_i, pressure outside the capillary in the interstitium; σ, a reflection coefficient; π_c, oncotic pressure inside the capillary; and π_i, oncotic pressure in the interstitium. Although this equation looks different from Ohm's law of electricity, it really is analogous and includes terms for flow, resistance, and a gradient for flow.

Don't get lost in the terms, though, they all make sense if you think about them. Pressure in the capillary minus pressure in the interstitium drives edema formation. Similarly, oncotic pressure in the interstitium minus that of the capillary also drives edema formation. The reflection coefficient describes the ease with which proteins cross the capillary endothelium; if capillaries were completely impermeable to proteins, the reflection coefficient would be 1, and if they were completely permeable (leaked all proteins), it would be 0.

Figures 10.4 and 10.5 attempt to put together all that you've learned. Figure 10.4 models the cardiovascular system during cardiac arrest. During arrest, all pressures (the height of blood in each

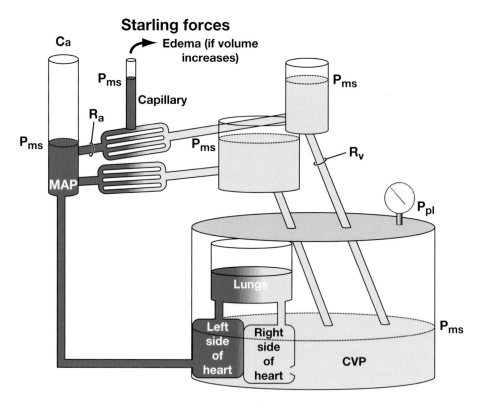

Figure 10.4. Cardiovascular System During Cardiac Arrest.

Ca denotes capacitance (or compliance) of the arterial system; CVP, central venous pressure; MAP, mean arterial pressure; P_{ms}, mean systemic pressure; P_{pl}, pulmonary pressure; P_{ra}, right atrial pressure; R_a, arterial resistance; R_v, venous resistance.

compartment) are at the same level. This is, by definition, the P_{ms} or circulatory arrest pressure, and it is depicted by the dotted line in each container. Figure 10.5 shows what happens when the heart is beating. Now, some of the blood in the large-capacity venous reservoir is pumped into the systemic arterial circulation (after transiting through the lungs). The pressure in the venous reservoir decreases, and the pressure in the arterial compartment increases. Because each compartment has a different compliance (or capacitance—either term will suffice), the decrease in venous pressure below P_{ms} is less than the increase in arterial pressure above P_{ms}.

This model places the smaller pulmonary circulation within its own pressure chamber (ie, the thorax, which also contains the heart). By doing so, it explains interventricular dependence (both the right and left sides of the heart are confined within the pericardium) and

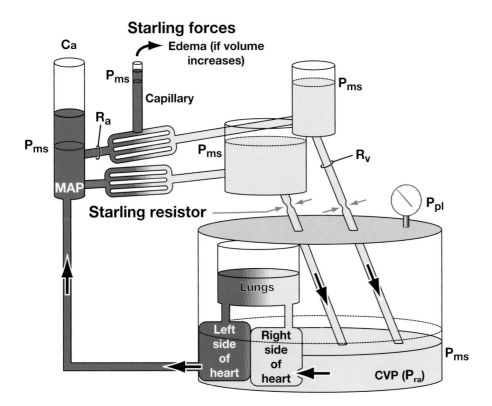

Figure 10.5. Cardiovascular System During Cardiac Activity.

The black arrows show direction of blood flow. The green arrows indicate Starling resistors. See Figure 10.4 legend for abbreviated terms.

shows how the large veins draining into the central circulation and thorax are subject to collapse, forming Starling (variable) resistors, when the thorax is under negative pressure (eg, spontaneous ventilation during inspiration). Note that each of the 2 parallel systemic circulatory paths shown have along their length a container labeled "P_{ms}." These containers represent the unique point in each systemic circulatory path where, as Starling said, the pressure neither rises nor falls during cardiac activity or arrest.

Another feature of this model is capillary overflow, which represents edema formation when total blood volume is increased. Note that capillary edema will not occur simply as a result of cardiac arrest alone, without a volume increase.

Finally, there is a practical consequence to this model. If we wanted to have a measure of how "full" the cardiovascular system is, we couldn't do better than P_{ms}, which gives us the ratio of stressed blood volume to cardiovascular compliance. This is more reflective of how full or empty the cardiovascular system is than the absolute blood volume alone (absolute blood volume always demands the qualifier, "How big is the patient?"). P_{ms} is not sensitive to the size of the patient because it has already corrected for that, and as we've noted previously, P_{ms} is not sensitive to how well or how poorly the heart functions.

That's all fine and good, but how do we measure P_{ms} without doing something as dramatic as Starling's stopping of the heart? The answer is simple—find the unique crossover point in the systemic circulation where the blood pressure is always at P_{ms} and measure it there. Where is that crossover point? It is the postcapillary venules and veins. Fortunately, venous pressures and resistances are very small, so the discrepancies when measuring pressure a few centimeters closer or further from the capillaries are trivial. Similarly, measurement of P_{ms} in a hand vein, foot vein, or upper arm vein doesn't make much difference.

Each systemic vein empties into a common final pathway, the right atrium. In the steady state, no significant disequilibrium is maintained between pressures in parallel veins because a "backward" pressure equilibration occurs from the right atrium into each circulatory path that drains into it. What about valves, don't they prevent backward equilibration from occurring? The answer, both theoretically and empirically, is no. Remember, an open valve cannot maintain a pressure gradient, and most venous valves remain open in the steady state because they are draining blood continuously. That's why intravenous anesthetic drugs don't linger in the peripheral veins before making their way into the central circulation—they make the trip right away. We also know this from compressing an arm or a leg proximal (closer to the chest) to a venous measurement site. When we do this, an immediate step-change in pressure is observed in the more distal (further from the chest) vein.

Finally, if we hypothesize that peripheral venous pressure is, in fact, the same as P_{ms}, we should see that it is unchanged during cardiac arrest. From the figure depicted at the end of Chapter 9 (Down But Not Out—Circulatory Arrest Pressures), you can see that it does not change.

QUESTIONS AND ANSWERS

Questions

10.1 Why doesn't acute tamponade cause peripheral edema?

10.2 Does the heart normally pressurize or depressurize the systemic capillaries?

Extra credit An insurance salesman knocks on a woman's door and asks how many kids she has. She says, "Three." He wants to know their ages. She thinks he's being too nosy and devises a riddle to make him work for the answer. She tells him that the product of their ages is 36 (all ages are whole numbers). He wants more information. She tells him that the sum of their ages is the same number as the neighbor's street address. The salesman scales the fence to see the neighbor's address and then returns and wants more information. She says, "My oldest child plays the piano." He tells her the 3 ages. What are they? (Adapted from Flannery S, Flannery D. In code: a mathematical journey. New York: Workman Publishing Company; 2001. p. 13–16. Used with permission.)

Answers

10.1 The clue to this answer is the term "acute." In a patient with a normal blood volume, mean systemic pressure (about 15 mm Hg) is lower than average systemic capillary pressure (about 25 mm Hg). Acute cardiac tamponade causes heart failure by filling the pericardium with fluid. As the heart fails, flow through the vasculature decreases, and the pressure gradients between the aorta and the right atrium also decrease. Thus, the pressure in the aorta decreases and the pressure in the right atrium increases. In the event of complete heart standstill, all pressures will equalize at mean systemic pressure. Because the systemic capillaries start at a pressure of 25 mm Hg, their pressure will decrease, not increase, and the capillaries will not leak or cause edema formation. In contrast, during chronic heart failure, the body compensates by retaining fluid and increasing blood volume. This greater volume causes mean systemic pressure to increase, eventually equaling or exceeding normal capillary pressure. As the heart continues to fail, peripheral edema occurs.

10.2 As is evident from the preceding answer, the heart normally pressurizes the systemic capillaries relative to circulatory arrest pressure (mean systemic pressure).

Extra credit The children are 2, 2, and 9 years old. The key to solving this problem is to recognize that the solution lies not just in algebra but also in the use of information. Let's call the children's ages A, B, and C. The salesman learns first that $A \times B \times C = 36$. This restricts the assortment of ages to the following possibilities: 1/1/36; 1/2/18; 1/4/9; 3/3/4; 2/2/9; 2/3/6; or 1/6/6. Next, the salesman learns that the sum of their ages is equal to a street address. Importantly, we don't know that address, but the fact that his knowledge of the address still doesn't allow him to answer means that at least 2 possible combinations of ages must sum to the same number. The only candidates are 2/2/9 and 1/6/6 (both sum to 13).The final statement, "My oldest child plays the piano," is not a random fact; like most statements in riddles, it conveys necessary information. The telling clue in the statement has nothing to do with the piano, however; the woman is indicating that she has an oldest child (single, not plural). That rules out 1/6/6 and leaves only 2/2/9.

· 11 ·

OXYGEN AND THE GRADIENTS
OF LIFE

IF YOU WERE INVITED into the operating room when a patient was undergoing deep hypothermic circulatory arrest (see Chapter 9 [Down But Not Out—Circulatory Arrest Pressures]), you would have a very hard time determining whether the patient was still alive. None of the vital signs would be looking all that vital. The patient would have no physiologically meaningful blood pressure (only the mean systemic pressure of about 15 mm Hg throughout the cardiovascular system), no pulse or heart rate, a body temperature of 18°C, and no respiration or even cardiopulmonary bypass circulation during the arrest phase. Nonetheless, the anesthesia team would expect the patient to recover from this state of suspended animation after being placed back on bypass and rewarmed; eventually, the patient would be separated from bypass with the heart beating on its own. Now here's a not-so-rhetorical question: physiologically, what is the difference between a patient undergoing deep hypothermic circulatory arrest and another patient who has died and cooled to the same temperature?

The answer resides inside the cells. During hypothermic arrest, physiologic functions of whole-organ systems are temporarily arrested, but the cells are still busy. To be sure, cellular metabolism is also slowed (that's the whole rationale of this technique—to quiet brain metabolism 7-fold so that it can tolerate a lack of circulation and oxygen for about 7 times longer), but it's not completely stopped. One difference between the hypothermic-arrest patient and the dead patient is that the former has live cells and the latter has dead cells. And furthermore, one of the differences between live cells and dead cells is that live cells maintain certain important gradients across their membranes. Another difference is that dead cells have no metabolism.

We often refer to cellular metabolism as "respiration," and we measure it by calculating how much oxygen is being used. We also use the term respiration to mean visible breathing ("ventilation"). Hypothermic circulatory arrest is one of those situations where the 2 terms are obviously separable. This brings us to oxygen. Why do we define cellular metabolism in terms of oxygen consumption? What's so special about oxygen that life not only depends on it but is in part defined by it?

To answer that question, we'll go back to England in the early 1960s. In addition to everything else going on in England during that time, an eccentric scientist named Peter Mitchell decided to put forward a hypothesis about what oxygen did in the mitochondria to drive metabolism. As you might gather from Figure 11.1, Peter Mitchell wasn't quite as popular as the Beatles, but he did have his own enduring effect.

Here is what was already known at the time. As the breakdown products of foods are metabolized in the citric acid (tricarboxylic acid) cycle, electron donors are generated. These donors (reducing equivalents) are reduced nicotinamide adenine dinucleotide (NADH) and reduced flavin adenine dinucleotide ($FADH_2$), and they travel to the matrix of the mitochondria, where they discharge their electrons at the top of an energy cascade (the *electron transport chain*) on the inner mitochondrial membrane.

Mitchell proposed a hypothesis that linked oxygen to life. He suggested that as electrons in the matrix are handed off between successive cytochromes, the energy generated is used to pump protons (H^+) across the inner mitochondrial membrane, forming a local pH gradient. If nature abhors a vacuum (see Chapter 1 [Pressure and Its Measurement]), it abhors a gradient even more. The proton gradient requires energy to establish and waits for an opportunity to dissipate. The best place for the gradient to discharge is through complicated proteins (ATPases) on the inner mitochondrial membrane. These proteins look a bit like doorknobs, with a central canal through which the

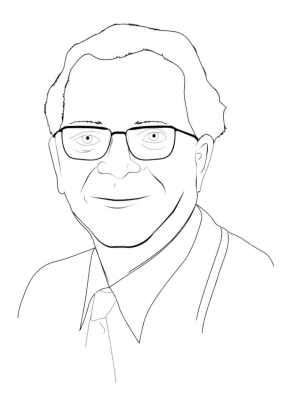

Figure 11.1. Peter Mitchell (1920-1992), originator of the chemiosmotic hypothesis.

protons pass back into the inner mitochondrial space. As the protons flow through the ATPases, the energy released is captured and used by the ATPases to generate adenosine triphosphate (ATP) from adenosine diphosphate (ADP) and inorganic phosphate.

Peter Mitchell called this model the *chemiosmotic hypothesis*, and it promptly aroused the derision of his colleagues. Not to worry, though, his idea has withstood the test of time, and it is now, in fact, textbook dogma. Mitchell also was awarded the 1978 Nobel Prize in chemistry for his insight. You'll find his name on the rafters of the Plummer Medical Library at Mayo Clinic—along with Vesalius and Harvey.

So where does oxygen fit into all of this? Oxygen has 2 characteristics that enable everything in the scenario above to work: 1) it readily diffuses from the atmosphere into the cells (thanks to all of the mechanisms of cardiopulmonary physiology that you have been studying); and 2) it is strongly "oxidizing," ie, it attracts electrons to itself. When a candle burns in the presence of oxygen, a high-energy substrate gives up electrons to oxygen (releasing water and carbon dioxide)—so, too, is it with our cells. Only when oxygen is at the end of the electron transport chain, along the inner mitochondrial membrane, do electrons cascade down that chain. When electrons get to the end of the chain, they combine with oxygen in a process that converts oxygen to water. That's where the oxygen goes, and that's why we constantly need more of it. Unfortunately, no other molecule that we know of can do exactly the same thing and function as a substitute for oxygen. Like Peter Mitchell, oxygen is one of a kind.

Figure 11.2 shows a schematic pathway for oxygen as it diffuses from a blood vessel into adjacent tissue and then into a mitochondrion. As you'll see in Chapter 12 (The Two Doctors Fick), this transport of oxygen through the blood and then down a partial pressure gradient can be described quantitatively by 2 separate concepts, both named after Dr Fick.

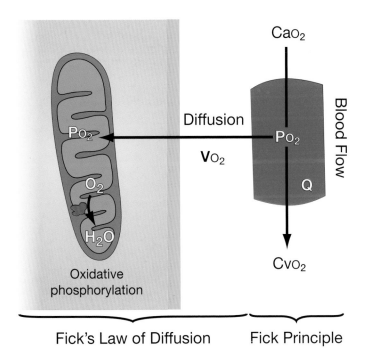

Figure 11.2. Schematic Pathway for Diffusion of Oxygen. Oxygen moves from a blood vessel, through adjacent tissue, and into a mitochondrion. Cao_2 denotes arterial oxygen content; Cvo_2, venous oxygen content; H_2O, water; Po_2, partial pressure of oxygen; Q, blood flow; Vo_2, oxygen consumption.

QUESTIONS AND ANSWERS

Questions

11.1 If a new molecule was discovered that could replace oxygen in animal respiration, what characteristics would it need?

11.2 Describe the "chemiosmotic hypothesis" of Peter Mitchell.

Extra credit In the mid 1970s, NASA's Viking expedition landed a probe on the surface of Mars and began to search for evidence of life in soil samples. It failed to find any. What kinds of tests do you think were performed?

THE TWO DOCTORS FICK

IT'S NO ACCIDENT THAT some scientists have made more than one important discovery in their lifetime. They have what you might call "systematic luck." Adolph Fick (1829–1901) was successful in several different fields—he has an eponymous law describing the diffusion of solutes and gases (1855), developed a method for calculating cardiac output (1870), and even made the first suggestion for contact lenses (1888).

For the sake of accuracy, and to make this brief discussion less confusing, I need to point out that we often confuse the "Fick principle" with "Fick's law of diffusion." They are not the same, although they were both put forward by the same Dr Fick. Ironically, Fick borrowed heavily from already known physical laws when he first described both his law of diffusion and his principle.

Let's take Fick's law of diffusion first, since it came first. Because Fick was trained initially as a mathematician and a physicist, it was natural that he would take a physicist's view of physiology. In fact, in the nineteenth century, he was one of the first scientists to do so. Borrowing from Ohm's law of electricity, Fick applied concepts of diffusion and transfer across a resistance to formulate a law of diffusion that could be applied to gas or solute transfer across a membrane. Whether we are talking about transfer across the alveolar-capillary membrane or across a dialysis membrane, the concept is the same. The terms in Fick's law of diffusion are a little

Answers

11.1 Such a molecule would have to be of sufficiently low density to allow ventilation without excess work of breathing. It would have to be nontoxic and relatively inert to body tissues. It would have to be readily diffusible across the alveolar-capillary membrane and the peripheral tissue membranes. It would have to bind to hemoglobin with the same degree of cooperativity as oxygen (ie, loading easily at lung partial pressures and unloading easily in the peripheral tissues), or it would need to be sufficiently soluble in the liquid fraction of blood to provide adequate mass transport to the tissues. Finally, it would have to support electron transport through the mitochondrial cytochrome chains by serving as an "electron sink" and be reduced to a nontoxic product after the terminal redox reaction. With this long list of functional requirements in mind, it's not surprising that we haven't found a substitute for oxygen in the maintenance of vertebrate life.

11.2 Simply put, Mitchell hypothesized that a proton pump is powered by electrons cascading down to ever lower levels of energy along an electron transport chain within the inner mitochondrial membrane. This pump establishes a proton (pH) gradient across the membrane. When discharged (like a battery), the potential energy of the proton gradient is converted to chemical energy and powers the conversion of inorganic phosphate group and ADP to high-energy ATP.

Extra credit In addition to searching for organic chemicals (which were not found), scientists searched for evidence of redox reactions, based on the assumption that biologic activity of any kind would require metabolic activity. An initial positive result from a labeled-release redox assay caused some to speculate that life had been found. However, the scientists recognized that the same result would be obtained if Martian soil contained nonorganic oxidizing materials. In 2008, the Phoenix lander discovered such material in the Martian soil, in the form of perchlorate salts.

more complicated than those of Ohm's law (ie, voltage, resistance, and current), but the concept is similar—you have 1) a transfer rate, 2) a resistance, and 3) a gradient:

$$Q = K(P_1 - P_2) \times S/t$$

where Q denotes diffusion rate; K, a diffusion coefficient (determined by membrane material, as well as solubility and molecular weight of the crossing molecule); $P_1 - P_2$, the diffusion gradient across the membrane (determined by partial pressures of the molecule on each side of the membrane); S, surface area of the membrane; and t, thickness of the membrane. If you consider the terms S, t, and K to all be components of resistance, you'll appreciate that Fick's law is really just a restatement of Ohm's law of electricity, only applied to diffusion.

Now let's consider the Fick principle. In 1870, Fick put forward an ingeniously simple method for measuring cardiac output. On the basis of another physical law (the law of conservation of mass), he understood that, in the steady state, the difference between the amount of oxygen going into a tissue bed minus that leaving the tissue bed must be equal to the oxygen consumed. With a little reworking, this became the Fick principle:

Cardiac output = O_2 consumption/(arterial O_2 – venous O_2).

To rephrase this by using terms that you're more likely to encounter in anesthesiology:

$$CO = Vo_2/(a-v\ Do_2)$$

where CO denotes cardiac output; Vo_2, oxygen consumption; and a–v Do_2, the difference between arterial and venous oxygen content. Please note that "a–v Do_2" is very different from the "$AaDo_2$" that we met on Mount Everest (Chapter 2 [Atmospheric and Alveolar Pressures]); that alveolar-arterial gradient for oxygen is a partial pressure gradient. Here, the arterial-venous oxygen difference measures oxygen *content*, not partial pressure. Oxygen content is the concentration of oxygen in a blood sample, and it is directly proportional to the total number of oxygen molecules in that sample. In contrast, partial pressure is related to the total number of molecules in a sample in a more complicated way. The oxyhemoglobin dissociation curve, which plots oxygen content (or percent saturation) versus partial pressure of oxygen, is sigmoidal, not linear.

The quantitative definition of arterial oxygen content is as follows:

$$Cao_2 = 1.37 \times [Hgb]\%Sat + 0.0031 \, Pao_2$$

where Cao_2 is arterial oxygen content and $[Hgb]\%Sat$ is the product of hemoglobin concentration and percent oxygen saturation. If you work out the stoichiometry of the coefficient 1.37 (knowing the molecular weight of hemoglobin, the fact that 4 molecules of oxygen bind to each molecule of hemoglobin, and using a little help from Avogadro), you will arrive at a coefficient of 1.39, not 1.37. Practically, it doesn't matter. Theoretically, the reason why 1.37 is used is because hemoglobin is never completely saturated (ie, not every hemoglobin molecule is bound to 4 oxygen molecules); thus, the smaller number accounts for the inevitable inclusion of a few aberrant hemoglobin species that can't bind 4 oxygen molecules.

To see if you understand the difference between content and partial pressure, try solving the following problem. You have 2 sealed containers, each containing 5 mL of blood from the same patient. One has a Po_2 of 100 mm Hg, the other has a Po_2 of 27 mm Hg. After mixing the samples together into one sealed container, what is the resulting Po_2? The answer is 40 to 45 mm Hg, which is 75% saturated with oxygen. Remember—contents (or saturations), not partial pressures, are additive.

Now, let's revisit the diffusion schematic (Figure 12.1) that you first saw in Chapter 11. You should be able to see that the Fick principle applies to calculations about the transport of oxygen in the blood (including its mass disappearance into the tissue), whereas Fick's law applies to the diffusion of oxygen from the blood to the cytochrome electron transport chain on the inner mitochondrial membrane.

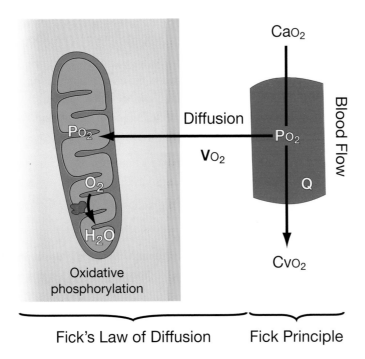

Figure 12.1. Schematic Pathway for Diffusion of Oxygen.
Oxygen moves from a blood vessel, through adjacent tissue, and into a mitochondrion. Cao_2 denotes arterial oxygen content; Cvo_2, venous oxygen content; H_2O, water; Po_2, partial pressure of oxygen; Q, blood flow; Vo_2, oxygen consumption.

QUESTIONS AND ANSWERS

Questions

12.1 Describe the difference between the Fick principle and Fick's law of diffusion. Write an equation that describes each.

12.2 If you were designing an extracorporeal membrane oxygenator, how would Fick's 2 concepts inform your strategy?

Extra credit You are blindfolded and breathing from a scuba tank in the center of an air-evacuated room when a large, dense, cold object is placed next to you without touching you. No air is available to circulate between you and the object. You can't see, yet you know where the object is because you feel colder on that side. Why is that? Can Fick's law of diffusion be invoked in the explanation, even in a vacuum (when the upstream element can't sense the downstream "pressure" corresponding to a transfer gradient through a medium)?

Answers

12.1 The Fick principle applies the law of conservation of mass to blood flow. In the case of measuring cardiac output, a quantity of dissolved oxygen (or a quantity of cold saline) is added to the bloodstream, and measurements are taken at a different point downstream. The quantity-versus-time profile of oxygen (or temperature) can be used to estimate blood flow. The same principle is applied to oxygen delivery, consumption, and return (of unconsumed oxygen) in the systemic circulation. The relevant formula, using oxygen content, is $CO = Vo_2 / (a - v \, Do_2)$, where CO denotes cardiac output; Vo_2, oxygen consumption; and a–v Do_2, the difference between arterial and venous oxygen content.

Fick's law of diffusion applies a principle similar to Ohm's law of electricity to the mass transport of substances across a membrane. Both Ohm's law and Fick's law relate 3 variables: 1) a gradient of the transported substance (either electrons or molecules); 2) a resistance (either within a wire or across a membrane) against the gradient; and 3) the corresponding current or flow. In the case of Fick's law, the relevant equation is $Q = K(P_1 - P_2) \times S/t$, where Q denotes diffusion rate; K, a diffusion coefficient (determined by membrane material, as well as solubility and molecular weight of the crossing molecule); $P_1 - P_2$, the diffusion gradient across the membrane (determined by partial pressures of the molecule on each side of the membrane); S, surface area of the membrane; and t, thickness of the membrane.

12.2 Fick's law of diffusion would suggest a blood oxygenating membrane that has a large surface area (S), small thickness (t), low diffusion coefficient (K; meaning that oxygen and carbon dioxide are readily soluble in the membrane and pass through it easily), and a large diffusion gradient $(P_1 - P_2)$ across the membrane. This last requirement would call for a high partial pressure of oxygen and a low partial pressure of carbon dioxide on the machine side of the membrane. The Fick principle would suggest maintaining a high carrying capacity for oxygen in the blood perfusing the oxygenator, as well as high blood flow through the oxygenator. Both would ensure an adequate delivery of oxygen to the peripheral tissues.

Extra credit Although Fick's law of diffusion describes solute or gas gradients in a medium, there is no medium here for the heat to move through, only airless space. Nevertheless, the key to this question is to understand that heat is a quantity and cold is only the absence of heat. With that perspective in mind, remember that your body is a source of heat and that your body radiates heat outward in all directions. (Of the 4 usual mechanisms of heat transfer [evaporation, conduction, convection, and radiation], only radiation is applicable here.) Similarly, the walls of the room contain a certain amount of heat, and they also radiate heat in all directions, including toward you. Because your body is warmer than the walls, the net transfer of heat is away from you and into the walls, equally in all directions, if you are in the middle of the room.

Now consider the cold object placed next to you. Remember to think of yourself as being warmer than the object, rather than it being colder than you (again, heat is a real physical entity, whereas cold is only the absence of heat). You will radiate heat toward the object and it will radiate very little heat toward you, less heat than that radiated by the surrounding walls. The net transfer of heat between you and your surroundings becomes asymmetric. You lose considerably more heat than you gain from the side near the cold object, and the temperature sensors in your skin detect that asymmetry.

By analogy, wind chill factor was first measured at an Antarctic research station by comparing the differential freezing rates of closed cans of beans. One was placed in the wind and one was in a shelter, shielded from the wind but at the same outdoor temperature. Both cans of beans radiated heat outward into the cold surroundings, and both heated up the air surrounding them. In the case of the wind-exposed can, air currents swept away layers of warmer air as they formed, resulting in a larger temperature gradient between the can and its surroundings and faster heat loss. This mechanism only makes sense if you think in terms of heat transfer, rather than of "cold transfer."

· 13 ·

A BREATH OF FRESH AIR—
VENTILATION

THE *SINE QUA NON* of ventilation is arterial carbon dioxide. If you want to know about ventilation, just check the Pa_{CO_2}. If it is low or normal, ventilation is fine, thank you—regardless of any other parameter, including respiratory rate, tidal volume, or dead space ratio. However, if Pa_{CO_2} is high, then alveolar ventilation (V_A) is impaired (relative to the carbon dioxide load being presented to the lungs). Another way of expressing this relationship is with a simple equation:

$$Pa_{CO_2} = K(V_{CO_2}/V_A)$$

where K denotes a constant; V_{CO_2}, whole-body CO_2 production; and V_A, alveolar ventilation. Figure 13.1 shows the equation expressed graphically.

V_A can also be calculated with a simple equation:

$$V_A = fV_T(1 - V_{DS}/V_T)$$

where f denotes respiratory rate (frequency); V_T, tidal volume; and V_{DS}, dead space volume. "Dead space" volume (V_{DS}) is the volume within the patient's airways (or within a breathing circuit) that is being ventilated to-and-fro with fresh gas and the patient's "old" lung gas, but no alveolar gas exchange is occurring. Total

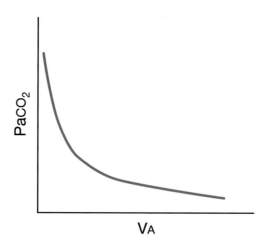

Figure 13.1. Relationship Between Alveolar Ventilation (V_A) and Arterial CO_2.

ventilation, often expressed as liters per minute (ie, minute ventilation [V_E]), is the sum of V_A and V_{DS}. Later on, you'll see that there are 2 different kinds of dead space ventilation, anatomic dead space and physiologic dead space.

In a conventional breathing circuit, dead space ends at the Y-shaped junction of the inspiratory and expiratory arms of the circuit and the endotracheal tube (Figure 13.2A). On the machine side of that junction, the inspiratory and expiratory limbs see only fresh inspired or expired gas, respectively, but not both. The endotracheal tube, in contrast, sees inspired and expired gases but does not contain gas exchange surfaces, and thus it contributes to dead space. The same is true of the trachea, mainstem bronchi, and multiple generations of conducting airways down to the alveoli. At the level of the alveoli, however, true gas exchange occurs at the alveolar-capillary membrane, so alveolar spaces are not considered dead space (Figure 13.2B).

You should know 2 other things about ventilation. One is the Bohr equation, which estimates the ratio of dead space to tidal volume:

$$V_{DS}/V_T = (Pa_{CO_2} - Pet_{CO_2})/Pa_{CO_2}$$

where V_{DS} denotes dead space volume; V_T, tidal volume; Pa_{CO_2}, partial pressure of arterial CO_2; and Pet_{CO_2}, partial pressure of end-tidal CO_2. This equation was derived by the early twentieth century

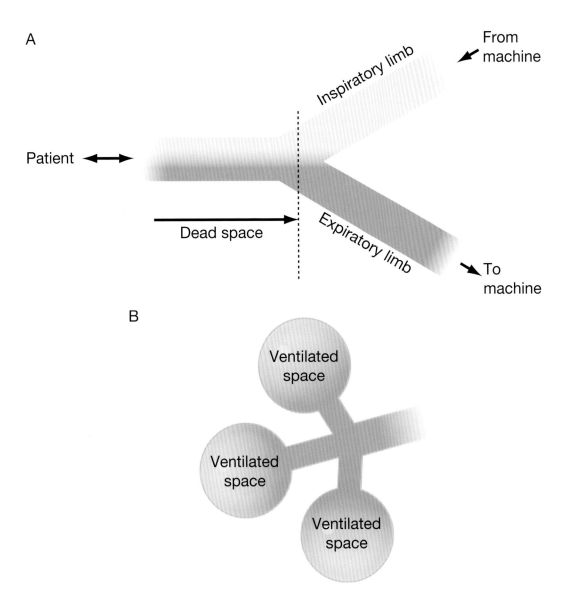

Figure 13.2. Anatomic Dead Space.

A, Dead space ends at the Y-shaped junction of the inspiratory and expiratory arms of the circuit and the endotracheal tube. B, Alveolar spaces do not contribute to dead space because gas exchange occurs at the alveolar-capillary membrane.

Danish respiratory physiologist, Christian Bohr. (Extra credit: Who was Christian Bohr's son?)

Keep in mind that the Bohr equation estimates *physiologic* dead space, not anatomic dead space. To estimate *anatomic* dead space, a single-breath nitrogen washout curve must be generated (Figure 13.3). This is also termed the *Fowler Method*.

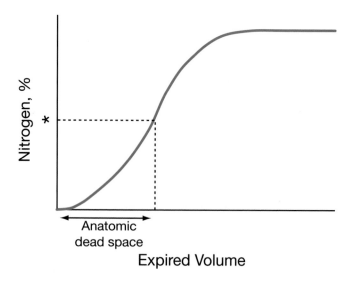

Figure 13.3. A Single-Breath Nitrogen Washout Curve (Fowler Method).
The asterisk indicates half maximal nitrogen content, and the corresponding expired volume indicates the anatomic dead space.

In this method, the subject takes a breath of 100% oxygen to total lung capacity and then exhales into a nitrogen monitor. The first gas seen by the monitor is pure oxygen from the anatomic dead space. It is followed by a mixture of oxygen and nitrogen from conducting airways and then by a nitrogen plateau, which represents gas from exchanging areas of the lungs. The anatomic dead space accounts for the first and approximately half of the second of these 3 phases. Or, more simply, the anatomic dead space is estimated as the expired volume that coincides with half maximal nitrogen content.

The second thing that you may want to know about ventilation is the effect of gravity on the distribution of ventilation within the lung. As you'll see in subsequent topics, this has implications for the matching of ventilation to perfusion in both normal and diseased lungs, as well as during one-lung ventilation for open-chest surgical procedures.

Figure 13.4A shows a compliance curve for alveoli in different elevations within the upright lung, extending from the base to the apex. Remember that compliance is defined as the change in volume divided by change in pressure ($\Delta V/\Delta P$ or dV/dP), so compliance in this figure is the slope of the sigmoid curve at any point.

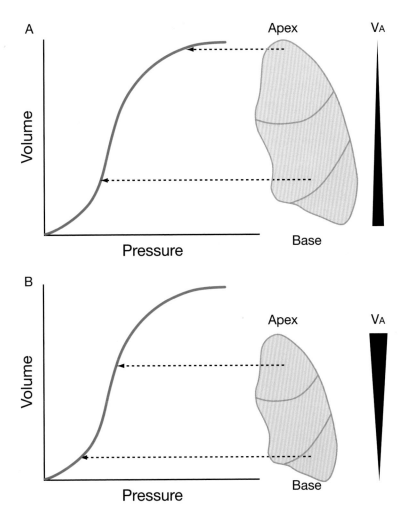

Figure 13.4. Compliance Curve for Alveoli in an Upright Lung.
A, Normal state. B, Pneumothorax. Vᴀ denotes alveolar ventilation.

While it may be counterintuitive, the alveoli at the apex of the lung are ventilated less than those at the base. The reason for this is that the alveoli at the apex are on a less compliant portion of the curve—ie, they are already distended compared with those alveoli at the base.

With the introduction of a pneumothorax (eg, during surgical thoracotomy), the entire lung tends to settle down to a lower volume because it is no longer surrounded by negative intrapleural pressure. As this happens, the highest regions of lung become more compliant ("slide down" to the steeper portion of the curve), and the bottom regions of lung become less compliant (Figure 13.4B). This will cause a reversal in the distribution of ventilation within the lung.

QUESTIONS AND ANSWERS

Questions

13.1 The measured Pa_{CO_2} of a patient is 60 mm Hg. Normal Pa_{CO_2} is 40 mm Hg. What physiologic variables could explain the observed hypercapnia? What are the relevant equations?

13.2 In an upright lung, why is alveolar ventilation higher at the base than the apex?

13.3 What does a pneumothorax do to the distribution of ventilation in the upright lung? Why?

Extra credit What are the Seven Wonders of the Ancient World?

Answers

13.1 Sometimes an equation (or two) is worth a thousand words. First, $Pa_{CO_2} = K(V_{CO_2}/V_A)$, where K denotes a constant; V_{CO_2}, whole-body CO_2 production; and V_A, alveolar ventilation. Second, $V_A = fV_T(1 - V_{DS}/V_T)$, where f denotes respiratory rate (frequency); V_T, tidal volume; and V_{DS}, dead space volume. These 2 equations encompass virtually everything that affects arterial carbon dioxide.

This patient has an abnormally high Pa_{CO_2}, which could be caused by a change in any of the variables in those 2 equations. Elevated whole-body CO_2 production could occur from fever or sepsis. Decreased alveolar ventilation could result from decreased respiratory rate (eg, narcotic overdose), decreased tidal volume (eg, splinting and pain from rib fractures), or an increase in dead space volume (eg, pulmonary embolism causing part of the lung to be ventilated but not perfused; or breathing through a long hose).

13.2 Look at the lung compliance curve again (Figure 13.4A). The alveoli at the base work at smaller volumes than those at the apex because they are compressed by the weight of the lung above them. At first, this might suggest that alveoli at the base would receive *less* ventilation. However, the lower alveoli have greater compliance (graph to a steeper part of the compliance curve), meaning that for a given change in pressure during inspiration, a greater volume change will result compared with alveoli at the apex. In the apex, alveoli are not as compliant (graph to a less steep part of the compliance curve).

13.3 A pneumothorax reverses the relative values of ventilation. The introduction of air into the pleural space causes the lung to partially collapse because the negative pressure around the lung is compromised and the chest wall can no longer provide support. All alveoli shrink to smaller volumes. Look again at the compliance curve (Figure 13.4B). If all alveoli are functioning at smaller volumes, the alveoli at the apex now graph to a steeper part of the compliance curve than alveoli at the base. For every inspiratory pressure change, the alveoli at the apex will now have a greater volume change.

Extra credit In no particular order, they are 1) Statue of Zeus at Olympia; 2) Colossus at Rhodes; 3) Temple of Artemis at Ephesus; 4) Lighthouse at Alexandria; 5) Great Pyramid at Giza; 6) Mausoleum at Halicarnassus; and 7) Hanging Gardens of Babylon.

· 14 ·

PULMONARY FUNCTION TESTS

PULMONARY FUNCTION TESTS (PFTs) sort out the ability of the lungs to *ventilate* and *oxygenate*. Before going to the details, don't forget that a careful history is also a PFT. For example, a patient with the diagnosis of chronic obstructive pulmonary disease (COPD) is unlikely to have extubation fail at the end of a routine general anesthetic procedure if he does not need home oxygen therapy and golfs regularly. In contrast, a patient who has symptomatic dyspnea, even before induction of anesthesia, will likely have problems at the end of the procedure, regardless of the specific PFT findings.

Perhaps the most useful PFT measures arterial blood gas (ABG). If we consider the lungs to be a "black box," then the functional products of that black box are the P_{O_2}, P_{CO_2}, and pH of arterial blood. In fact, so long as those 3 parameters are within acceptable physiologic limits, we don't need to know much else about the lungs. Consider the extreme case of a patient on cardiopulmonary bypass—lungs aren't needed at all because the heart-lung machine removes CO_2 and adds O_2 to the blood. In other words, once we've established that the ABG is normal, it doesn't much matter whether pulmonary function is provided by a machine or is natural, nor do specific respiratory parameters (eg, tidal volume, respiratory rate, flow rate) matter as much as the end result of pulmonary function—the ABGs.

With just 3 bits of primary data (arterial pH, P_{CO_2}, and P_{O_2}), the ABG gives incisive information about acid-base status, ventilation, and oxygenation (Figure 14.1).

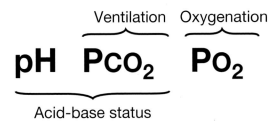

Figure 14.1. Pulmonary function status can be determined by arterial pH and blood gas pressures.

Pco_2 denotes partial pressure of CO_2; Po_2, partial pressure of O_2.

The simple algorithm described below can be used as a "quick and dirty" interpretation of ABGs; you can perform this in your head without using nomograms, computers, or even pencil and paper.

Step 1: Consider only the arterial pH, Pco_2, and Po_2. Most of the other numbers reported with an ABG are derived (calculated), not primarily measured. For example, the bicarbonate is calculated from the pH and Pco_2. It is all right to use the bicarbonate value or the base deficit number as rough markers of metabolic acidosis, but remember that they are calculated measures.

Step 2: Is the pH normal, acidotic, or alkalotic? Assume, for ease of calculation, that a normal arterial pH is 7.40.

Step 3: Is the Pco_2 normal, increased (indicating hypoventilation), or decreased (indicating hyperventilation)? Assume a normal arterial Pco_2 is 40 mm Hg.

Step 4: If the pH is abnormal, can Pco_2 alone account for the abnormality? Know the following rule of thumb: for every 10 mm Hg change in Pco_2, there is a corresponding change in pH of 0.08 in the opposite direction. Any deviation of pH from normal that can be traced to changes in Pco_2 is respiratory in origin. Any additional deviation from normal pH is assumed to be metabolic in origin.

Step 5: In a mixed acid-base disturbance with both respiratory and metabolic origins, the primary disorder alters the pH more than the compensatory disorder. For example, if a patient has a coincident metabolic acidosis and respiratory alkalosis (pH 7.36; Pco_2, 30 mm Hg), how do you know which is the primary

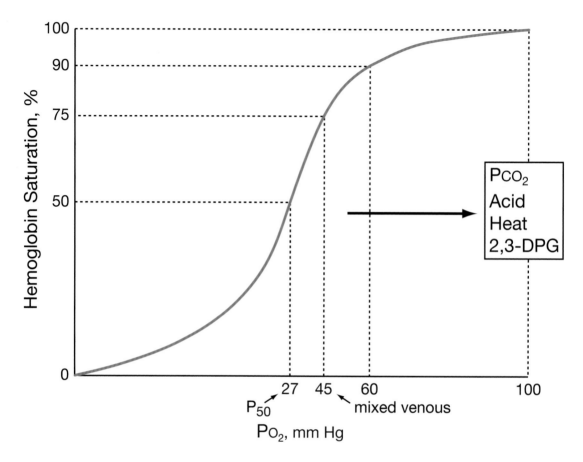

Figure 14.2. Oxyhemoglobin Dissociation Curve.

The curve is shifted to the right by increases in P_{CO_2}, acid, heat, or 2,3-diphosphoglycerate (2,3-DPG).

disorder? The P_{CO_2} of 30 mm Hg predicts a pH of 7.48 (see the rule of thumb in step 4), but the measured pH is acidotic. Thus, the metabolic acidosis "wins"—it must be the primary disorder, and the respiratory alkalosis must be the compensatory disorder.

Step 6: What is the P_{O_2}? Now that you know how to calculate an alveolar-arterial gradient, you can put numbers to the efficiency of lung oxygenation (Figure 14.2). As you learned in Chapter 2 (Atmospheric and Alveolar Pressures), the alveolar-arterial gradient indicates how well the lungs can oxygenate blood, independent of the level of alveolar ventilation. Because the alveolar air equation accounts for alveolar P_{CO_2}, any clinically significant gradient will be due to the other causes of hypoxemia (Box 14.1; see Chapter 2 for definition of terms).

Box 14.1. Physiologic Causes of Hypoxemia

Causes alveolar-arterial gradient
    Diffusion impairment
    Ventilation/perfusion (V/Q) mismatch
    Shunt
Does not cause alveolar-arterial gradient
    Hypoventilation
    Lowered F_{IO_2}
    Lowered P_B

The next type of PFT is probably already familiar to you. *Spirometry* is the measurement of inhaled and exhaled lung gas, as depicted in Figure 14.3 (relevant terms are defined in Table 14.1). Before considering each parameter, you should note that in spirometry, a "capacity" includes 2 or more "volumes." Also, note that residual

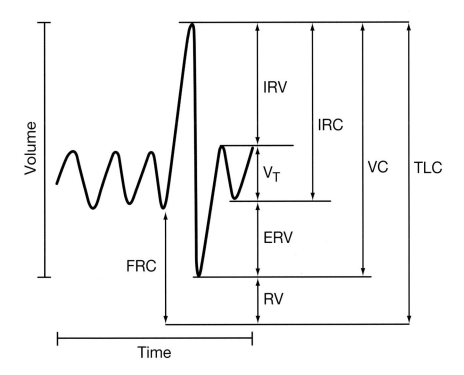

Figure 14.3. Spirogram.

(See Table 14.1 for definition of relevant terms and approximate normal values.)

Table 14.1. Normal Values for Spirometry

Term	Definition	Approximate Normal Values (70-kg man)
ERV	Expiratory reserve volume	…
FEF_{25-75}	Forced expiratory flow (in midvolume range)	4 L
FEV_1	Forced expiratory volume (in the first second)	4 L
FEV_1/FVC	Ratio of FEV_1 and FVC	80%
FRC	Functional residual capacity	3 L
IRC	Inspiratory reserve capacity	…
IRV	Inspiratory reserve volume	…
RV	Residual volume	2 L
TLC	Total lung capacity	7 L
VC (or FVC)	Vital capacity (or forced vital capacity)	5 L
V_T	Tidal volume	0.5 L

volume (RV) cannot be determined by the measurement of inhaled and exhaled gas volume alone. Either body plethysmography or gas dilution methods are needed to determine RV (and, therefore, to determine functional residual capacity or total lung capacity as well).

The next PFT is the *flow-volume loop* (Figure 14.4). Before looking at how the loop changes with pathologic conditions, you should be familiar with the axes of the graph. Note that the horizontal axis is inverted, with high volumes closer to the origin and low volumes further from the origin.

Figure 14.5 shows how the flow-volume loop changes with lung disease. With *obstructive* lung disease (eg, COPD, asthma), the lung volumes tend to shift to higher values, and there is a characteristic concavity in the expiratory phase. This concavity is caused by an effort-independent obstruction to flow in the mid ranges of expiration, and it is characteristic of either small-airway disease or bronchospasm. With *restrictive* lung disease (eg, kyphoscoliosis, morbid obesity), in contrast, the absolute volumes are shifted to lower values, and the expiratory phase demonstrates higher relative flows at a given lung volume.

Why does small-airway disease cause effort-independent obstruction? To answer that question, you'll need to know about *time constants*.

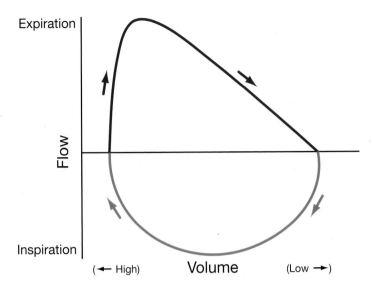

Figure 14.4.   Flow-Volume Loop.

Simply put, a time constant is an index of how fast something fills or empties, whether that something is an alveolus, a balloon, a blood vessel, a pharmacokinetic compartment, or a bathtub.

Let's consider the bathtub first (Figure 14.6). In nature, most things empty or fill in a nonlinear fashion. In a bathtub, the pressure

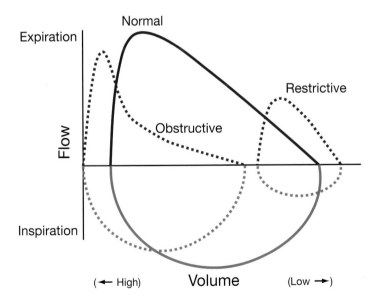

Figure 14.5.   Flow-Volume Loop With Obstructive or Restrictive Lung Disease.

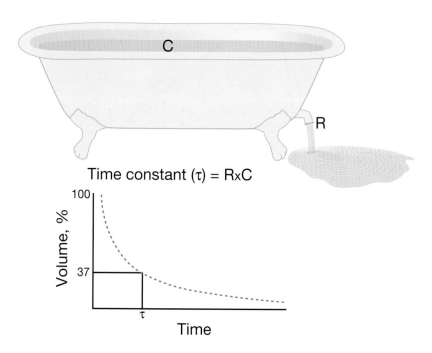

Figure 14.6. Definition of Time Constant.

As the bathtub drains, the pressure head above the drainage hole decreases and the flow rate decreases nonlinearly. The time constant is the time needed to empty 63% of the starting volume (or fill to 63% capacity [not shown]). C denotes capacitance (or compliance in a closed, expandable container); R, resistance; τ, time constant.

head above the drainage hole decreases as water drains, and the resulting flow rate decreases with time. The product of resistance (R) and capacitance or compliance (C) is the time constant (τ), which corresponds to the amount of time that it takes for the object either to fill to 63% capacity or empty 63% of its starting volume.

This concept is easily transferred to the case of alveolar filling and emptying (Figure 14.7). Instead of capacitance, though, the alveolus is considered to have a compliance. Fortunately, both start with the letter C, so we can use the same designation (R×C) for the time constant. You can see that the amount of time for the alveolus to empty also will be determined by the R and C values of its lung unit. Either a large R value or a large C value will contribute to a larger time constant and, therefore, a longer emptying time.

Patients who are on the emphysema end of the COPD spectrum have lung tissue destruction that results in overly compliant (large C)

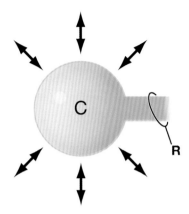

Figure 14.7. Alveolus Expanding and Contracting.
C denotes compliance; R, resistance.

alveoli. They breathe easier at higher absolute lung volumes because they are on a less compliant part of the lung distension curve and the C values are lower. In contrast, patients who are on the chronic-bronchitis end of the COPD spectrum and patients with asthma have no problem with large C values—instead, they have large R values (higher resistance to outflow). Like their emphysema counterparts, though, the time constant (RC) is still too large for efficient emptying.

Let's go back to the question about why small-airway disease causes effort-independent obstruction. In a nutshell, while the patient is straining his or her thorax in an effort to exhale more quickly (thereby decreasing C), the conducting airways are being compressed in the midexpiratory volume range, which results in a simultaneous increase in R. The net result is an unchanged time constant for emptying—air does not leave the lung any faster, despite the increased effort. By analogy, imagine that you are trying to force air as quickly as possible from an inflated balloon. However, as you squeeze the balloon harder, you simultaneously compress the neck of the balloon; thus, the outflow rate stays the same.

Let's apply these concepts to pathologic lung obstructions. There are 4 main types of obstructions: 1) fixed extrathoracic, 2) fixed intrathoracic, 3) variable extrathoracic, and 4) variable intrathoracic (Figure 14.8). Fixed obstructions, whether they are intrathoracic or extrathoracic, have the same effect on breathing. Variable

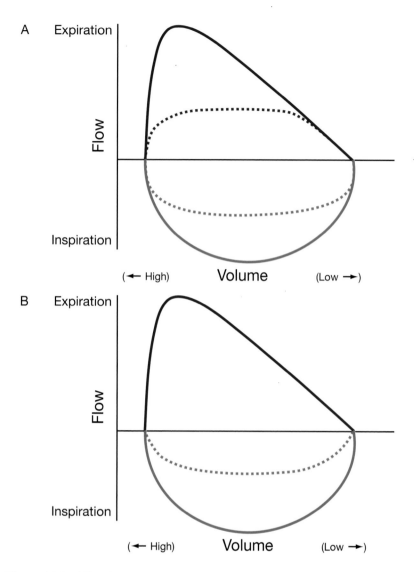

Figure 14.8. Flow-Volume Loop With Obstructive Lung Disease. A, Fixed obstruction. B, Variable extrathoracic obstruction.

extrathoracic obstructions do not interfere with expiration, but they do obstruct flow during inspiration because airway pressure inside of the obstructed segment decreases during inspiration and the airway tends to collapse. Variable intrathoracic obstructions have just the opposite effect. The site of obstruction is actually stented (held open) by negative intrathoracic pressure during inspiration, but the airway collapses from positive intrathoracic pressure during expiration.

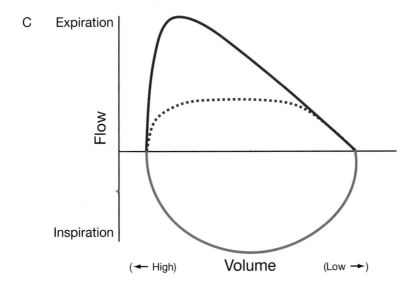

C   Expiration

Flow

Inspiration

(← High)   **Volume**   (Low →)

Figure 14.8. *Continued*

C, Variable intrathoracic obstruction.

Finally, the test measuring diffusing capacity of the lung for carbon monoxide (DLco) rounds out the list of commonly used PFTs.
You'll learn more about diffusing capacity and diffusion limitation
in Chapter 17 (Diffusion Limitation—Montana Style), but for now,
the basics of this test will suffice. DLco is measured and reported
in units of mL of carbon monoxide (CO) per mm Hg per minute.
An average normal value for an adult is about 30 mL CO per mm
Hg per minute. Diseases that result in decreased DLco include idio-
pathic pulmonary fibrosis and bleomycin toxicity. In fact, administration of bleomycin during prolonged courses of chemotherapy is
guided by serial DLco measurements.

CO is used to measure diffusing capacity because of its incredi-
bly high affinity for hemoglobin. Because CO so readily binds hemoglobin, the pulmonary blood acts as a sink for CO after it diffuses
across the alveolar capillary membrane. This prevents substantial
CO from building up "back pressure," which would interfere with
further CO diffusion across the lungs. As a result, the net transfer
of CO across the alveolar capillary membrane is dependent almost
exclusively on the diffusing capacity of the membrane (it does not
depend on pulmonary blood flow).

As you discovered in the discussion of *Fick's Law of Diffusion* (Chapter 12 [The Two Doctors Fick]), the transfer of a solute or gas across a membrane depends on the thickness, surface area, and the intrinsic solubility of the crossing molecule in the membrane. The transfer of a gas across a membrane is also a function of its partial pressure gradient. Highly blood-soluble gases like CO are considered *diffusion limited* across the lung, and less-soluble gases are considered *perfusion limited*. Less-soluble gases build up a substantial partial pressure in the blood; this opposes further diffusion of the gas from the alveolus to the blood. Such gases depend more on perfusion, which acts to remove the undissolved fraction of gas away from the alveoli, allowing further diffusion.

QUESTIONS AND ANSWERS

Questions

14.1 Interpret the following arterial blood gases (ABGs), measured for patients breathing room air at sea level.

Patient	pH	P_{CO_2}, mm Hg	P_{O_2}, mm Hg
1	7.40	40	100
2	7.32	50	100
3	7.48	30	100
4	7.25	30	60
5	7.25	55	45

14.2 Draw and label a spirometric tracing.

14.3 Draw a normal flow-volume loop. Superimpose a loop consistent with chronic obstructive lung disease.

14.4 Draw a normal flow-volume loop. Superimpose a loop consistent with a variable intrathoracic obstruction.

Answers

14.1

Patient	Arterial Blood Parameters	Diagnosis	Comment
1	Normal pH Normal CO_2 Normal O_2	Normal ABG	...
2	Acidotic Increased CO_2 Normal O_2	Pure respiratory acidosis	Hypercapnia accounts completely for the altered pH.
3	Alkalotic Decreased CO_2 Normal O_2	Pure respiratory alkalosis	Hypocapnia accounts completely for the altered pH.
4	Acidotic Hypocapnic Hypoxemic	Primary acidosis, with partial respiratory compensation	A low P_{CO_2} should cause alkalosis, but the pH is acidotic in spite of the low P_{CO_2}. Remember that the primary pH disorder "wins" and moves the pH further than the compensatory effort. A P_{O_2} of 60 mm Hg is substantially lower than that predicted by the alveolar air equation (using a P_{CO_2} value of 30 mm Hg), so this patient has intrinsic lung disease causing hypoxemia.
5	Acidotic Increased CO_2 Hypoxemic	Mixed respiratory/metabolic acidosis	Hypercapnia does not entirely account for a pH of 7.25. Even though the P_{CO_2} is elevated, the alveolar air equation does not predict an O_2 level as low as 45 mm Hg, so this patient also has intrinsic lung disease.

14.2 Please review Figure 14.3.

14.3 Please review Figure 14.5.

14.4 Please review Figure 14.8C. A variable intrathoracic obstruction will collapse with the high intrathoracic pressures generated during expiration, but the obstructed area will be stented open by the negative intrathoracic pressures generated during inspiration.

· 15 ·

WHERE BREATH MEETS BLOOD—
LUNG PERFUSION

ARISTOTLE (FIGURE 15.1) LIKED to describe form in the context of function. In other words, he wasn't afraid of invoking teleology or "thinking from the end" in his descriptions of anatomy. If you were Aristotle's student (like Alexander the Great), you also would be taught to think about anatomy in terms of functional end points. In our era, though, teleologic explanations have been frowned on as if they were logical errors—they are the sort of "why" questions that science shouldn't ask. That's beginning to change, though, as molecular biologists and genomics experts begin to talk more to their physiology colleagues and as they begin to make sense of what gene expression means at the level of the whole organism. For example, without looking to the "end" (ie, the physiologic or functional requirements of the whole organism), it is difficult to make sense of the integrated patterns of gene expression that affect the survival of the organism. Unless the functional consequences of gene expression are understood, it is hard to argue that gene expression is understood. We inevitably come back to asking and answering "why" questions. Aristotle would be proud.

Let's come back to the respiratory system. By analogy to what we just observed about thinking in terms of functional requirements, we might say that the pulmonary circulation is a low-resistance, low-pressure, high-flow system because its primary function is to

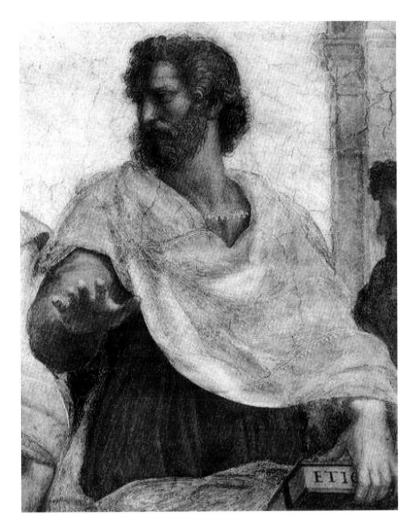

Figure 15.1.   Detail of Aristotle.

(From Raffaello Sanzio da Urbino [Raphael], artist. "The School of Athens" [painting]; 1510. Located at: The Vatican, Rome.)

oxygenate blood. For that reason, pulmonary circulation is different from systemic circulation. Because resistance is lower in pulmonary circulation, pressures across the pulmonary vascular bed also are substantially lower (systolic pressure is 120 mm Hg in the aorta but only 25 mm Hg in the pulmonary artery).

In a teleologic sense, why is the pulmonary system a low-pressure system? If you think about it, an oxygenator system that matches air to blood must meet numerous requirements. You would need a large surface area for air and blood to come into contact with each other, especially since we're mammals with a high metabolic requirement and therefore a high oxygen requirement. You would want that contact surface to be thin (remember Fick's Law of Diffusion) but not so thin that membranes rupture easily. You would want to prevent the membrane from drying out, which is why you might want to enclose it within the body to keep it moist.

An efficient system includes inherently low resistance. This allows the entire cardiac output to flow through without high-pressure areas, thereby diminishing the danger of rupturing thin gas-exchange surfaces. Nevertheless, rupture can occur in pathologic conditions like pulmonary edema at high altitude or from mitral valve insufficiency. Only a slight increase in transmural pressure within the pulmonary capillaries can tip the Starling forces in favor of edema. That's just a consequence of having efficient gas-exchange surfaces in the lung.

One other consequence of low resistance is that the pulmonary circulation is unusually susceptible to the effects of gravity. If you remember the discussion about gravity and the cerebral circulation, gravity affects local transmural pressures (inside minus outside pressures at each segment of a blood vessel) but has no effect on perfusion pressure (inlet minus outlet pressure). No substantial part of the cerebral circulation collapses in the head-up position because it is held open by the rigid cranium and the architecture of the venous sinuses. Pulmonary circulation is different. There is less "stenting open" of pulmonary capillaries, and they are therefore more likely to partially or fully collapse when transmural pressure becomes negative.

The diagram in Figure 15.2 is probably already familiar to you, but let's revisit it to be sure that you understand how gravity affects pulmonary blood flow. In the upright lung, transmural pressure at the apex is less than that at the base, owing to the differences in hydrostatic pressure as you move from the top of the lung to the bottom.

In a mechanically ventilated patient or in a patient with very low blood pressure, zone 1 conditions can occur, resulting in the complete collapse of some apical pulmonary capillaries. In zone 2, a "choke point" occurs where the alveolar pressure midway through

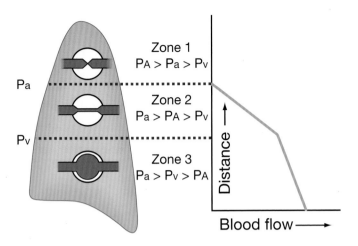

Figure 15.2. Supposed Behavior of Small Vessels in 3 Zones of the Lung With Regional Differences in Blood Flow.

The lung is divided into zones according to relative pressures. PA denotes alveolar pressure; Pa, pulmonary artery pressure; Pv, pulmonary venous pressure. (Adapted from West JB, Dollery CT, Naimark A. Distribution of blood flow in isolated lung: relation to vascular and alveolar pressures. J Appl Physiol. 1964;19[4]:713-24. Used with permission.)

the pulmonary circulation is higher than the far downstream venous pressures. This has been called a "Starling resistor" or a "vascular waterfall." In zone 3, the far downstream venous pressure exceeds alveolar pressure, and alveolar pressure is correspondingly less relevant to resistance and flow.

If you look at the graph on the right side of Figure 15.2, pulmonary blood flow is represented as a function of distance from the base of the lung. In zone 1 conditions, blood flow is absent. In zone 2 conditions, Pa increases as you move from the apex toward the base (because of the simple effect of hydrostatic pressure increasing relative to heart level), although PA, a gas pressure, is essentially unchanged within that small vertical distance. As a consequence, the difference between Pa and PA increases as you move down zone 2, and blood flow also increases.

How about zone 3? Why should blood flow increase in a zone where Pv is the downstream pressure, when both Pa and Pv increase at the same rate down that zone? The reason is that transmural vascular pressure increases as you move from the apex toward the base, and the increase in transmural pressure causes *recruitment* of otherwise closed capillaries and *distention* of those already opened. This, in turn, causes a decrease in local pulmonary vascular resistance.

As you might guess, pulmonary circulation also is affected during spaceflight. In a weightless environment, the distribution of pulmonary blood flow and ventilation becomes more homogeneous, so ventilation-perfusion matching and oxygenation are slightly improved.

Have a look at Figure 15.3. You already know from the discussion of ventilation that the apical alveoli of the healthy, upright lung are less ventilated than those at the base (remember why?). Now include the vertical distribution of blood flow (Q) next to alveolar ventilation (VA), and you'll see that while both VA and Q increase from apex to base, Q increases more. Therefore, the VA/Q ratio *decreases* as you move from the apex to the base of the lung. Where would you expect to see the highest local P_{AO_2}? If you were a tubercle bacillus, where would you want to live within the lung? I would want to reside and multiply within the apical alveoli because that's where the local P_{AO_2} is highest.

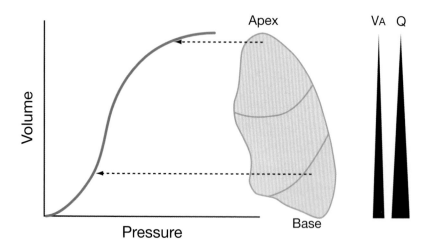

Figure 15.3. Compliance Curve for Alveoli in an Upright Lung.

Q denotes vertical distribution of blood flow; VA, alveolar ventilation.

QUESTIONS AND ANSWERS

Questions

15.1 What happens to the ventilation-perfusion ratio (V_A/Q ratio) as you move from the apex down to the base of the upright lung? Why

15.2 What is the content of oxygen (ie, the volume percent [vol%] of oxygen) in atmospheric air? What is the oxygen content (vol%) of arterial blood (Ca_{O_2}) in a healthy subject at sea level?

15.3 Describe West's zones of the lung and the main factors that govern pulmonary blood flow in each of those zones.

Extra credit What happens to West's lung zones with the application of positive end-expiratory pressure (PEEP)? What happens to the zones during a negative inspiratory effort against a closed glottis?

Answers

15.1 The V_A/Q ratio is higher at the apex than at the base. Both ventilation and perfusion increase from the apex down to the base of the upright lung, but perfusion increases at a faster rate. Consequently, local Pa_{O_2} is also higher at the apex than the base.

15.2 The atmosphere is 21% oxygen; thus, the content of oxygen in atmospheric air is 21 mL/dL or 21 vol%. Use the following equation from Chapter 12: $Ca_{O_2} = 1.37 \times [Hgb]\%Sat + 0.0031$ Pa_{O_2}, where Ca_{O_2} is arterial oxygen content and $[Hgb]\%Sat$ is the product of hemoglobin concentration and percent oxygen saturation (assume a normal hemoglobin level of approximately 15 g/dL and 100% saturation). Ca_{O_2} is approximately 20 vol%. Note that the content of oxygen in the atmosphere is almost identical to the content of oxygen in arterial blood.

15.3 You should be able to reproduce Figure 15.2. Pulmonary blood flow is absent in zone 1 because alveolar pressure exceeds arterial pressure and the pulmonary vessels are closed in that zone. Zone 2 is where, in theory, blood flow corresponds to the gradient between the upstream (arterial) pressure and an intermediate (alveolar) pressure that exists outside of the collapsible intermediate portions of the vessel (ie, a "vascular waterfall" or "Starling resistor"). According to the theory of the Starling resistor, far downstream (venous) pressure is irrelevant to flow. Blood flow in zone 3 increases as you move downward within that zone because of pulmonary vessel recruitment and distension.

Extra credit With the application of PEEP, P_A increases throughout all lung zones, but Pa and Pv remain the same. This will cause the boundaries between the zones to move downward, expanding zone 1 at the expense of zone 3. Just the opposite occurs with an inspiratory effort against a closed glottis. In that case, P_A decreases throughout the lung and the boundaries between lung zones move upward, expanding zone 3 at the expense of zone 1.

· 16 ·

BIRD BRAINS AND BIRD BREATH

JUST WHEN WE HUMANS think that we've achieved something remarkable (like climbing Mount Everest without supplemental oxygen), the animal kingdom trumps us. The bar-headed goose (Figure 16.1), for example, actually flies over the summit of Mount Everest during its annual trans-Himalayan migration. The summit of Everest is 29,028 feet, which means that a bar-headed goose manages to maintain vigorous exercise in the thin air of 30,000 feet. Try setting your treadmill to that level!

Like mammals, birds are warm-blooded animals (homeotherms). This means that they are metabolically active, even in the coldest or highest environments, and they have to maintain a constant flow of oxygen to the brain if they want to remain neurologically intact and still enjoy the view. To keep oxygen flowing at high altitudes, the bird must massively hyperventilate. One consequence of hyperventilation, though, is severe hypocapnia and respiratory alkalosis. Remember the blood gas and alveolar air sample from humans on the summit of Everest? The $P_{A}CO_2$ was an astonishing 7 mm Hg! This is an example of one form of homeostasis taking priority over another. The preservation of PaO_2 is apparently more important physiologically than the preservation of $PaCO_2$ or acid-base status.

Regardless of competing needs, though, it is still remarkable that these birds can achieve high enough oxygenation to support life (and exercise) at such extraordinary altitudes. That said, birds do have an

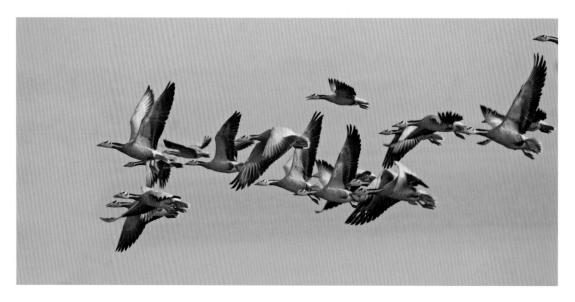

Figure 16.1.   Bar-Headed Goose.

(Copyright Rahul Sachdev. Used with permission.)

unfair advantage over us—their lungs use a system of ventilation/perfusion matching that is more efficient than that of the mammalian to-and-fro alveolar lungs. How does this work? To begin with, the bird lung is invested with a series of hollow air channels, not dead-end alveoli. These air channels are connected to a network of thoracic air sacs, which are each like a bellows. When the air sacs contract and relax in coordination, they force inspired air through the air channels in an almost continuous, unidirectional flow. Furthermore, the air channels contact the pulmonary vessels in an architectural array that looks suspiciously like a *countercurrent exchange* device.

You may remember from basic physiology that countercurrent exchange occurs in the loops of Henle to concentrate urine. Countercurrent exchange is also engineered into blood infusion devices to rapidly warm intravenous fluid or blood for patients with extensive hemorrhage. Whatever its specific application, countercurrent exchange takes advantage of the concept that 2 media will exchange properties (eg, solutes, heat, moisture) between themselves more efficiently if they are very close to each other and if they are flowing in opposite (antiparallel) directions. The concept is the same, no matter what is being exchanged.

There is, however, a poor cousin to countercurrent exchange, termed *crosscurrent exchange*. In a crosscurrent arrangement, one material divides into multiple parallel branches, and each of these branches crosses over the other material at multiple points. Although crosscurrent exchange looks superficially similar, it is not quite as efficient as countercurrent exchange. Still, it beats an alveolar to-and-fro matching of ventilation to perfusion. For a while, there was controversy about whether the bird lung used crosscurrent or countercurrent gas exchange. With some concepts, a picture is worth a thousand words, so before considering the answer, have a look at Figure 16.2.

Notice that the crosscurrent exchange system has blood with the same Po_2 crossing the air channel at each point, whereas the countercurrent system allows the blood to remain in contact with the air channel throughout the length of the vessel. This arrangement allows blood to be oxygenated to the highest air channel Po_2 without being admixed with poorly saturated blood.

Now, anatomy aside, how could you determine which system is used by the bird? An ingenious answer to that question was put forward by the comparative physiologists Johannes Piiper and Peter Scheid in 1972. Because the efficiency of gas exchange in a true countercurrent system depends on the relative direction of the 2 flows, they reasoned that reversing the direction of flow in 1 of the 2 media (either air or blood) would impair gas exchange and result in lower Pao_2. In contrast, reversing the direction of flow of either

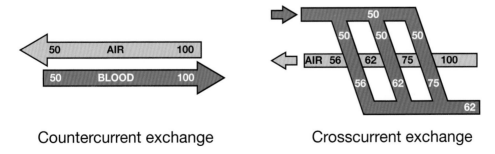

Countercurrent exchange   Crosscurrent exchange

Figure 16.2.   Bird Lung Controversy.

Numbers indicate percent oxygen saturation.

ventilation or perfusion in a crosscurrent system would not change its efficiency and therefore would not change Pao$_2$.

When Piiper and Scheid performed the experiment on an anesthetized bird (reversing the unidirectional flow of artificial ventilation through its lungs), the Pao$_2$ did not change significantly. That experiment provided physiologic evidence for crosscurrent gas exchange, and the mechanism was later confirmed by anatomic evidence. Thus, the bird lung is better than ours, but it still is not quite perfect.

The same experiment could be performed with membrane oxygenators used for cardiopulmonary bypass. Some of these devices have an array of tiny air tubes that allow passage of machine-controlled air next to adjacent tubes carrying blood, and oxygen and carbon dioxide are exchanged in this network. Even without opening and dissecting the oxygenator box, you could perform a Piiper-Scheid–type experiment to see if the gas exchange used crosscurrent or countercurrent exchange.

QUESTIONS AND ANSWERS

Questions

16.1 Describe the difference between crosscurrent and countercurrent exchange. Which is more efficient? Why?

16.2 How are the arteries and veins that perfuse the legs of a stork arranged so it doesn't lose too much heat when standing in cold water? How about in a dolphin flipper that radiates heat when the dolphin needs to cool down but also conserves heat when the dolphin swims in chilly water? What allows a dolphin to switch between "radiate" and "conserve" strategies without having to grow a different type of flipper each time?

Extra credit A fair coin is flipped 49 times and yields heads for all 49 tosses. What is the probability that it will come up heads on the fiftieth toss?

Answers

16.1 In a countercurrent arrangement, the materials being exchanged flow in antiparallel directions while maintaining close contact. In a crosscurrent arrangement, one material divides into multiple parallel branches, and each of these branches crosses over the other material at multiple points. The countercurrent exchange is more efficient because it maintains a greater partial pressure gradient for gas transfer over a longer interface distance.

16.2 For both examples, an efficient heat exchanger is established through a countercurrent vascular supply to the limb. Anatomically, blood vessels are arranged with warmer arterial blood running in close proximity and antiparallel to cooler venous blood. Physiologically, this arrangement retains core body heat at the expense of cooler limbs. In the case of the dolphin flipper, venous return from the limb can take different routes back to the heart: 1) along the surface of the flipper and away from the central artery (which radiates heat) or 2) alongside the central artery (which acts as a countercurrent heat exchanger and conserves core heat). The venous return route is determined by the actions of vascular sphincters that respond to temperature changes in the surrounding water.

Extra credit The probability of heads is 50%. For a truly fair coin, each event is independent of the sequence of preceding events. "Luck" neither builds up nor dissipates in a series of independent events. The probability of flipping 50 heads in a row is extremely small ($1/2^{50}$), but even if 49 heads have been achieved by chance, the remaining coin toss is not affected by what came before.

· 17 ·

DIFFUSION LIMITATION—
MONTANA STYLE

THE PATHWAY OF OXYGEN through the body can be described as a series of 2 leaps and a ride. The leaps are the diffusion of oxygen across the alveolar-capillary membrane and then the peripheral tissue membranes, whereas the ride is the convective transport of oxygen in the blood. Any transport process will have its choke points and limitations. In the case of oxygen, the constraints can take 1 of 2 forms, *perfusion limitation* or *diffusion limitation*.

One word of caution—for diffusion limitation, remember to think in terms of *partial pressure* of oxygen, not oxygen content. When we consider diffusion of a gas, we're really talking about the movement of that gas along a partial pressure gradient. For diffusion limitation to occur, it doesn't matter how many total gas molecules get moved from one place to another. Instead, what matters is whether the partial pressures on both sides of a membrane come to an equilibrium because that's what determines whether a gradient exists.

How does this fold into our previous discussion of Fick's Law of Diffusion (Chapter 12)? Remember that Fick's Law relates the mass transfer of molecules across a membrane to the pressure gradient across the membrane: $Q = K[P_1 - P_2] \times S/t$. (See Chapter 12 for the definition of all variables.) Specifically, the rate of oxygen transport across the alveolar-capillary membrane is directly proportional to the surface area of the membrane and to the partial pressure gradient of oxygen across the membrane (ΔP), but it is inversely related to the thickness of the membrane. In addition, the diffusion rate is directly proportional to the diffusion coefficient (K), and K is proportional to the ratio of solubility of the molecule in the membrane to the square root of the molecular weight of that molecule.

In the case where the resistance of the membrane is high enough to prevent pressure equilibration from occurring (ie, the ΔP term never becomes zero), then we have diffusion limitation and Fick's Law predicts the rate of mass transfer of molecules across the barrier. In contrast, if resistance across the membrane is so low that the partial pressure gradient across the membrane disappears and equilibration occurs, then Fick's Law is no longer relevant. In that case, the mass transfer of molecules into the blood is determined only by the total rate of blood flow, not by what Fick's Law predicts about the membrane resistance. This is perfusion limitation. So Fick's Law is relevant in conditions of diffusion limitation but not during conditions of perfusion limitation.

Have a look at Figure 17.1. If we want to make an analogy between the movement of oxygen from its partial pressure in the alveolus (P_{AO_2}) to its final partial pressure in the pulmonary capillary (Pa_{O_2}), then we might consider the loading of cattle onto a moving boxcar. The question before us is not how many cows get loaded (mass transfer); rather, does the density of cows in the boxcar ever reach the density of cows on the loading platform before the boxcar moves on? In other words, does Pa_{O_2} ever equal P_{AO_2} before the red blood cell moves away from the alveolus?

To answer that question, let's look at 4 conditions that could prevent equilibration from occurring. First, if the boxcar arrives at the loading platform completely empty, it will take longer to fill. This is analogous to having a very low mixed venous P_{O_2}. Second, a train moving too fast is analogous to high cardiac output (Qt). Third, a very narrow boxcar door corresponds to an alveolar-capillary membrane diffusion barrier (eg, pulmonary fibrosis, bleomycin toxicity, pulmonary edema). Fourth, a very big boxcar is analogous to very high solubility of the gas in blood.

Most of these points are intuitive, except for the last one. At first blush, a very large boxcar would seem advantageous for loading cattle onto the train quickly. But remember, we're not concerned

A

B

How full is the "empty" boxcar? (PvO₂)
How fast is the train moving? (Qt)
How wide is the door? (DLCO)
How big is the boxcar? (O₂ solubility)

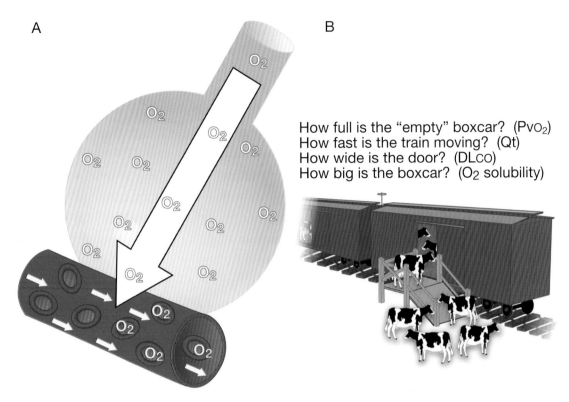

Figure 17.1. Diffusion Equilibrium.

A, Movement of oxygen from the alveolus to a blood vessel. B, Transfer of cows onto a moving boxcar.

here with the absolute number of cattle loaded—instead, we want to know whether the same density of cows can be attained inside the boxcar as outside before the train moves on. If you remember back to atmospheric pressure and Mount Everest (Chapter 2 [Atmospheric and Alveolar Pressures]), I asked how diffusion limitation could occur in such fit subjects as Everest climbers. The wrong answer is that the P_{IO_2} is so low. By itself, low P_{IO_2} will decrease partial pressure of oxygen throughout the entire body, will decrease mass transfer of oxygen molecules from the lungs to the blood, and therefore will cause hypoxia, but low P_{IO_2} alone will not cause diffusion limitation across the alveolar-capillary membrane. Although diffusion limitation can cause hypoxia, the converse is not necessarily true.

In the case of the Everest climbers, hypoxia caused a reflex hyperventilation mediated by the carotid bodies. This in turn caused an impressive respiratory alkalosis and left-shifting of the oxyhemoglobin dissociation curve. One way to think about the oxyhemoglobin dissociation curve is that it relates partial pressure to oxygen content (or saturation). That's the definition of solubility. A left-shifted curve is equivalent to increased solubility of oxygen in blood, and that's analogous to a bigger boxcar. A bigger boxcar presents no impairment to the mass transfer of cows, but it does present a problem if your objective is to fill the boxcar completely in a limited amount of time.

In medical school, you learned about a peculiar pulmonary function test called "diffusing capacity" or "diffusing capacity of the lung for carbon monoxide" (DLco). Why use carbon monoxide to study diffusion limitation? The reason is that the solubility of carbon monoxide in blood is extraordinarily high (2 orders of magnitude higher than that of oxygen). This means that for carbon monoxide, the boxcar is enormous and thus very hard to completely fill in a short time. If you want to study the diffusing capacity of the alveolar-capillary membrane, then you had better be sure that the gas you're using is limited by diffusion across the membrane, rather than by something else. Whether we're studying anesthetic gases, oxygen, or carbon monoxide, the following guideline applies: the more soluble a gas is in blood, the more likely it is to be diffusion limited, and the less soluble it is, the more likely it is to be perfusion limited.

Let's go back to the cows. If you're interested in testing how wide the boxcar door is in terms of its maximal limit for allowing cattle through, you'll want to be sure that the boxcar is so big that it never completely fills in the time allowed for your test. One way to think about perfusion limitation is in terms of full boxcars. If each car on the train can be quickly and easily filled with cows (ie, no diffusion limitation), then the limiting factor for mass transfer of cattle will be proportional to the speed of the train and the number and size of boxcars. However, if none of the boxcars ever fill during their passage across the loading platform, then the mass transport of cattle won't be helped by making the boxcars bigger or the train faster.

Physiologists who study the equilibration of gases across membranes think in terms of the ratio of gas solubilities—comparing solubility in the fluid on the other side of the membrane with solubility in the membrane itself. In addition to everything else you've just learned, the more soluble a gas is in a membrane, the easier it can diffuse across it. If the ratio is high, the gas is more likely to be diffusion limited. If it's low, it's more likely to be perfusion limited.

QUESTIONS AND ANSWERS

Questions

17.1 Describe the difference between diffusion limitation and perfusion limitation.

17.2 What factors can result in diffusion limitation?

17.3 Why is carbon monoxide a diffusion-limited gas in the lung?

Extra credit You have a series of fuses, each of which burns at varying rates (sometimes faster, sometimes slower during the burn), but all take precisely 30 minutes to burn from end to end. Using those fuses, how can you measure exactly 45 minutes?

Answers

17.1 Diffusion limitation occurs when a gas (usually oxygen) fails to reach partial pressure equilibration across a membrane (usually the alveolar-capillary membrane). Perfusion limitation occurs only when the partial pressure of a gas reaches equilibration across the membrane; in this case, the limiting factor for mass transport of the gas is the rate of blood flow. In diffusion limitation, blood flow is irrelevant because the blood leaving the lungs is not fully saturated with the gas.

17.2 Diffusion limitation occurs when there is a high resistance (R) to the transport of the gas across the membrane or a high degree of solubility (high capacitance [C]) of the gas in the medium on the other side of the membrane (or both). Analogous to the time constant (R×C) in an electrical circuit, a large R or a large C value (or both) will result in diffusion limitation because the time constant is large (ie, a longer time is needed for equilibration of the gas on either side of the membrane). Gases such as carbon monoxide, which are highly soluble in blood (high C value), are more likely to be diffusion limited than gases such as nitrous oxide, which are less soluble in blood.

17.3 Like oxygen, carbon monoxide binds to hemoglobin, but it actually binds with greater affinity than oxygen. As described above, hemoglobin in the blood has enormous capacity for carbon monoxide. This increases its equilibration time to the extent that equalization of partial pressures across the alveolar-capillary membrane never occurs.

Extra credit Make a circle out of one fuse and attach a straight fuse to a single point on the circle. Light the straight fuse and wait until both fuses are completely consumed. This will take exactly 45 minutes.

· 18 ·

MAN, MACHINE, AND HOMEOSTASIS

THE NINETEENTH CENTURY WAS a time of machines. The industrial revolution was in full swing, and the potential of using engineering solutions to solve human problems seemed limitless. Equally limitless were the possible analogies between machines and humans, often drawn to better understand human physiology.

One of the pioneers of physiology and experimental medicine during this period was the French physician Claude Bernard (Figure 18.1). In one sense, Bernard's timing was unfortunate because it coincided

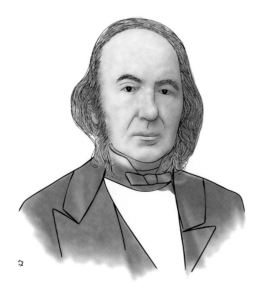

Figure 18.1.   French Physician Claude Bernard (1813-1878).

with (and was somewhat eclipsed by) the extraordinary work of Louis Pasteur in the new field of bacteriology. Nevertheless, Bernard lived in a time when very little was known about the mechanisms underlying physiologic findings, and he had ample access to clues garnered from observing machines. For a curious scientist, it was like being a kid locked in a candy store overnight.

Let's consider homeostasis, an example for which an engineered machine shed light on a fundamental principle of physiology. Homeostasis is simply the tendency of the body to maintain important physiologic variables (eg, heart rate, blood pressure, P_{ACO_2}) at constant, preset values. Although Bernard championed the *concept* of homeostasis, the term itself was not coined until the twentieth century by the Harvard physiologist Walter B. Cannon.

Take a look at the machine in Figure 18.2. It depicts a simplified mechanical governor that could be used to regulate the rotational

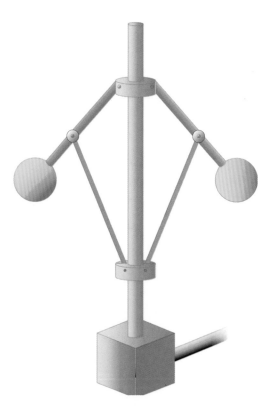

Figure 18.2. Simplified Mechanical Governor.

This device helps maintain constant rotational speed of steam engine shafts.

speed of a steam engine shaft. "Autoregulate" might be a more apt word because the governor performs without external help or guidance, provided it is designed and built properly. How does it work? As the steam engine shaft picks up speed, the rotating, weighted arms on the connected vertical shaft swing outward, producing a larger moment arm for rotation and slowing the turning shaft. As the shaft slows, the weighted arms fall back inward, reducing the moment arm, and allowing the shaft to turn faster. As it is with a spinning figure skater, the distance of the arms from the central axis affects turning speed. In addition, the levers attaching the weights to the central shaft are connected to a collar and rod (not shown) that opens and closes a throttle valve to control the supply of steam. This simple mechanism keeps the steam-driven shaft rotating at a remarkably constant speed.

It doesn't take much imagination to see an analogy between the mechanical governor and the autonomic nervous system. Both maintain specific variables at a constant set point through a process of feedback loops. A feedback loop schematic is pictured in Figure 18.3. There are 2 arms to the loop, an afferent (sensor) arm and an efferent (effector) arm. A central controller receives sensory information about the variable of interest and compares that value with the desired set point. If the values are discrepant (resulting in an "error,"

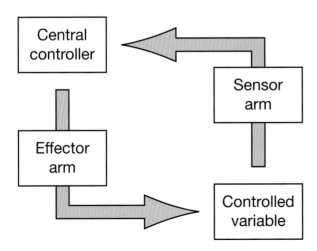

Figure 18.3. Feedback Loop.

The loop has an afferent (sensor) arm and an efferent (effector) arm.

in engineering parlance), the central controller effects a change in the variable through its effector limb.

Now let's look at a real example of autonomic feedback control of a physiologic variable: the carotid body chemoreceptor. Figure 18.4 depicts the way the carotid body functions in the afferent limb of a respiratory control loop. Remember that the *carotid body chemoreceptor* is not the same as the *carotid sinus baroreceptor*. The former senses blood gas values and controls ventilation. The latter senses arterial wall stretch and controls blood pressure by autonomic adjustment of the heart and blood vessels (see Chapter 1 [Pressure and its Measurement] for a more detailed discussion of the carotid sinus baroreceptor).

The carotid bodies are paired structures that are embedded in the wall of the carotid arteries. These structures have the highest mass-specific blood flow and the highest mass-specific oxygen

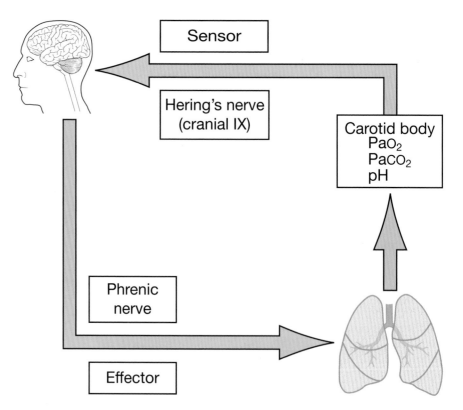

Figure 18.4. Carotid Body Feedback Loop.

consumption rate of any organ in the entire body, and they are involved in the process of monitoring properties of arterial blood. First, they sense Pa_{O_2}, not Ca_{O_2}, although the mechanism they use to determine the partial pressure of oxygen is unknown; in other words, they are sensitive to hypoxia but not anemia. Second, they are able to sense Pa_{CO_2} and arterial pH. Third, they can sense the rate of change in each variable (Pa_{O_2}, Pa_{CO_2}, and arterial pH). Fourth, the carotid bodies are invested with the biochemical apparatus necessary to make carbon monoxide as a byproduct of heme degradation. No one knows what function that serves, but it may provide a hint about how the carotid body senses Pa_{O_2}.

When arterial pH or Pa_{O_2} decrease or when Pa_{CO_2} increases, the carotid bodies sense that change and adjust the firing rate of the afferent nerves that connect to the brain stem. This in turn causes the brain stem respiratory control centers to adjust the traffic of nerve firing in the phrenic nerve, which controls diaphragm activity and ventilation. Respiratory acidosis, hypercarbia, or hypoxemia each can increase the firing rate of the phrenic nerve. Similarly, respiratory alkalosis, hypocarbia, or high Pa_{O_2} can decrease phrenic nerve activity.

In any autonomic control loop or negative feedback loop, the system is defined in part by the variable *gain*, which is calculated as follows:

Gain = Corrective Effort / Error

Like anything else in life, if a little bit of something is good, it doesn't necessarily mean that a lot is better. If the gain in a system is too high, a positive feedback cycle can be started. Positive feedback cycles (eg, bringing a microphone too close to a speaker) are inherently unstable. Thus, the autonomic nervous system uses negative feedback loops, not positive feedback loops. The former stabilize variables, whereas the latter destabilize them.

Nature does have some use for positive feedback, though; one example is when an explosion is created. The bombardier beetle (Figure 18.5) fends off aggressive predators by mixing a combination

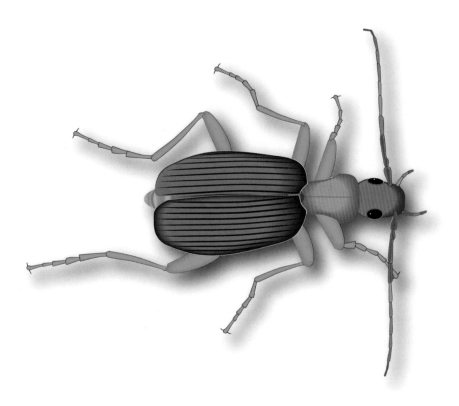

Figure 18.5. Bombardier Beetle.

of chemicals in a special chamber in its abdomen. This exothermic reaction feeds on itself and culminates in an explosion of hot, noxious chemicals that are sprayed onto the predator. Like any other positive feedback loop or "chain reaction," the process continues until its substrates are depleted and it is no longer self-sustaining.

QUESTIONS AND ANSWERS

Questions

18.1 Draw a basic feedback loop and describe its components.

18.2 Define *gain* in a feedback loop.

18.3 Why are positive feedback loops so rare in biological systems?

Extra credit What is the mechanism of death when a monkey is hit by a curare-tipped blow dart? (Hint: It's not asphyxia—you can't apply enough curare to a dart tip to paralyze the diaphragm).

Answers

18.1 Please review Figure 18.3. The loop has an afferent (sensor) arm and an efferent (effector) arm. Sensory information about the variable of interest is compared with the desired set point value. If the values are discrepant, a central controller effects a change in the variable through its effector limb.

18.2 *Gain* is the ratio of corrective effort to error.

18.3 Positive feedback loops are inherently unstable. They escalate their actions in an exponential "vicious" cycle, analogous to an explosion. Except in rare cases like the bombardier beetle, for which a true explosion of heated, noxious gases serves as a deterrent to predators, positive feedback loops generally are more destructive than useful.

Extra credit The extraocular muscles controlling the direction of the eyes are exquisitely sensitive to muscle relaxants. Even a small amount of curare causes weakness in these muscles and results in diplopia (double vision), which in turn causes a loss of depth perception. Death typically occurs after a monkey misjudges distance when leaping between branches and falls from a tree.

· 19 ·

PUTTING IT ALL TOGETHER—
MANNED SPACE FLIGHT

AT THE BEGINNING OF this book, you learned that there are 3 main sources of pressure in physiology: atmospheric, hydrostatic, and mechanical. One of the benefits of studying odd applications or environments is that it forces us to reconsider what we already know about physiology. When the envelope is pushed by high altitude, extreme exercise, the duress of disease states, or by being under water, physiologists have opportunities to see whether theory holds up against reality. In the twenty-first century, another unusual opportunity beckons: manned space flight to Mars (Figure 19.1). Although no firm date has been set, the National Aeronautics and Space Administration (NASA) has already drawn up preliminary plans for a manned space flight to Mars or perhaps to one of its moons, Phobos or Deimos.

Unless a feasible method to generate "artificial gravity" is developed (such as in-flight rotation of all or part of the spacecraft), the astronauts on board will experience about 888 days of weightlessness or reduced gravity during a Mars mission. Even if the flights have the benefit of rotational gravity, the time spent on the Martian surface (approximately 1.5 years) will test the limits of human adaptation to gravitational change, given that Mars has only 38% of the g force of Earth.

What does this mean physiologically? Let's take the case of prolonged exposure to zero-gravity conditions during a nonrotational

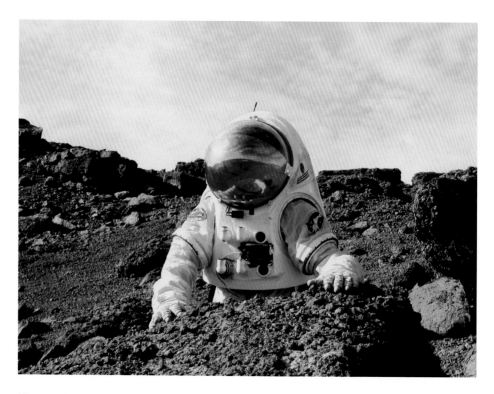

Figure 19.1.   Artwork depicting an astronaut on Mars.

(Adapted from Lee P. Field Report, August 8, 2001: Haughton Crater [Internet]. Moffett Field [CA]: Mars Institute, NASA Ames Research Center. Photo NASA Haughton-Mars Project; Report No. HMP-2001-0808. Available from: http://www.marsonearth.org/interactive/reports/2001/HMP-sr-080801.html. Used with permission.)

interplanetary flight. If the NASA spacecraft is pressurized to the equivalent of 1 atmosphere, then the atmospheric and alveolar pressures that we encountered in Chapter 2 will be unchanged. The alveolar air equation will still be relevant because the barometric pressure is 760 mm Hg. What about mechanical pressures generated by the heart, blood vessels, and the muscles of respiration? They will remain similarly unchanged, except for whatever atrophy or deconditioning occurs during the mission. Remember that the muscles of the cardiovascular system are smooth muscles, whereas the muscles of respiration are skeletal (or voluntary) muscles, even though they are under the control of the autonomic nervous system. (That's why you don't have to lay awake at night and concentrate on breathing, although you can consciously override autonomic ventilation and hold your breath or hyperventilate.)

One interesting and apparently intractable problem of reduced gravity is muscle wasting. Regardless of their exercise or diet regimens, astronauts lose muscle mass and muscle strength while aloft. They don't come bounding out of space shuttles right after returning from a mission—they can't stand without help because they're simply too weak and have orthostatic intolerance. Presumably, skeletal muscle wasting is caused partly because the astronauts' antigravity postural muscles aren't under constant use the same way they are at home. Hopefully, the skeletal muscles of respiration will not atrophy because they still will be constantly used and exercised. There are no iron lungs in space.

What about hydrostatic pressures? Here is where everything changes. Remember that hydrostatic pressure is determined by ρgh, where g is acceleration due to gravity. In weightless environments, $g=0$ by definition (thus, the term "zero-g"…. See, this isn't really rocket science, is it?). Without gravity, there is no possibility of a hydrostatic pressure gradient. What is the practical effect of losing the hydrostatic pressure gradient? Apparently, it has very little effect because astronauts seem to survive and their brains seem to be perfused just fine during exposure to weightless environments. This reconfirms what you've already been taught about cerebral perfusion pressure (inlet pressure minus outlet pressure; or mean arterial pressure minus right atrial pressure) being independent of gravity.

If you recall our discussion of giraffes, the circulatory system is a closed loop. This relieves the heart of the need to work against gravity; it just has to generate enough fluid energy to drive blood beyond the resistance of the blood vessels. In space, that point is no longer controversial. Remember that each point in a circulatory loop has its own transmural pressure (inside pressure minus outside pressure), and transmural pressure does depend on distance above or below the level of the heart. In a weightless environment, though, only the mechanical pressure generated by the heart contributes to transmural pressure. For example, when you examine cerebral circulation in weightlessness (Figure 19.2), you will have a mechanical pressure (P) curve and an intracranial pressure (ICP) component, but there will be no hydrostatic pressure (ρgh) line (see Chapter 4 [Doctor Dolittle Visits a Sitting Case]). This means that at any given

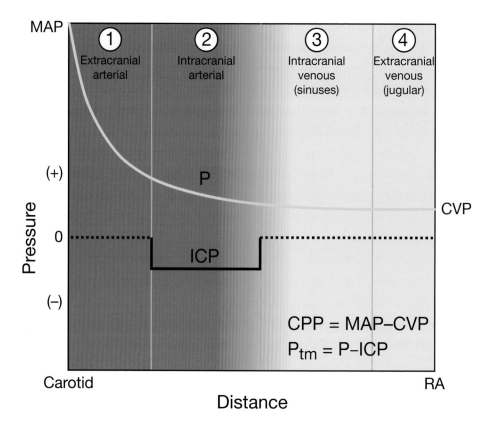

Figure 19.2. Difference Between Cerebral Perfusion Pressure and Local Transmural Pressure.

CPP denotes cerebral perfusion pressure; CVP, central venous pressure; ICP, intracranial pressure; MAP, mean arterial pressure; P, mechanical pressure generated by the heart; P_{tm}, transmural pressure; RA, right atrium. (Adapted from Munis JR, Lozada LJ. Giraffes, siphons, and Starling resistors: cerebral perfusion pressure revisited [editorial]. J Neurosurg Anesthesiol. 2000 Jul;12[3]:290-6. Used with permission.)

point in the cerebral circulation, the transmural pressure will be the simple sum of mechanically generated heart pressure (which decays as it flows through the resistance of the cerebral blood vessels) and intracranial pressure (only when the vessels are exposed to it).

If you've been paying attention, you'll know why I predict that giraffes will still have very high arterial blood pressure in space. The giraffe's cerebral perfusion pressure hasn't changed, nor has its cerebral vascular resistance changed. Only the distribution of transmural pressures along the cerebral circulatory path has changed, and those pressures are irrelevant to flow.

There is another physiologic challenge in space, however, and the concepts that you've learned in these chapters might make a very practical difference. One of the problems that astronauts experience is a decrease in total blood volume, which results in orthostatic intolerance upon returning to Earth. We don't know just how severe those alterations in volume will be during a prolonged space flight (eg, to Mars), but indications from other American and Russian missions suggest that they may be quite serious. Similar to the loss of skeletal muscle in spite of exercise, normal thirst mechanisms and the homeostatic feedback loops that you learned about in the previous chapter may be inadequate to maintain healthy hydration status.

It is unlikely that astronauts can or should be monitored with central venous pressure (CVP) lines during an extended mission. Such lines are maximally invasive, difficult to place, and dangerous to maintain for prolonged periods. The usefulness of CVP measurements in weightlessness also is unclear. Data from the space shuttle program indicate that CVP may rise, fall, or remain unchanged during the brief transition from 1 g to weightlessness.

One intriguing possibility for hydration status monitoring is the estimation of mean systemic pressure (P_{ms}). As you might remember, P_{ms} is the ratio of stressed blood volume to total vascular compliance; it is, therefore, a direct index of cardiovascular filling, independent of cardiac activity or central venous pressures. Fortunately, the estimation of P_{ms} is quite simple—it can be assessed by measuring the transmural pressure in any peripheral vein. This measurement is minimally invasive and accounts for hydrostatic pressure gradients on Earth or their absence in space. On Earth, the pressure transducer is placed at the level of the heart to neutralize the effect of gravity on the measurement. In space, the transducer can be placed anywhere.

The estimation of P_{ms} by peripheral venous pressure (Figure 19.3) may provide a simple way of monitoring the astronauts' hydration status in space and also may provide healthy target values, should intravenous hydration be necessary. Close attention to Starling's lessons from the nineteenth century may pay dividends in the twenty-first.

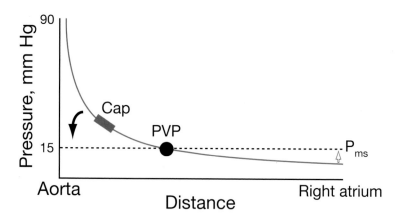

Figure 19.3. Blood Pressure Decay Curve.

The plot shows blood pressure as a function of distance from the aorta to the right atrium. During heart failure, the left side of the pressure decay curve decreases to converge with P_{ms} (black arrow), whereas the right side of the curve increases to converge with P_{ms} (white arrow). Cap denotes capillary pressure; P_{ms}, mean systemic pressure; PVP, peripheral venous pressure. (Adapted from Munis JR, Bhatia S, Lozada LJ. Peripheral venous pressure as a hemodynamic variable in neurosurgical patients. Anesth Analg. 2001 Jan;92[1]:172-9. Used with permission.)

QUESTIONS AND ANSWERS

Questions

19.1 When measuring peripheral venous pressure in a zero-*g* environment, why doesn't the position of the pressure transducer relative to the heart matter?

19.2 It's unlikely that any astronaut will undergo emergency brain surgery during space travel, but let's say that one does. If you remember from Chapter 4 (Doctor Dolittle Visits a Sitting Case), a perforation of a cerebral sinus or vein can cause venous air embolism (air sucked into the blood vessel) if the brain is elevated above the heart. Can venous air embolism occur in a zero-*g* environment?

Extra credit At the surface of the Earth, the theoretical maximal height of a water column sustained by a vacuum above the column is about 33 feet (equivalent to 1 atm of pressure). Nonetheless, giant sequoia trees can reach heights exceeding 300 feet, and they bring water from the roots to the highest leaves. A major mechanism for moving water through a plant is transpiration, which involves evaporative water loss from small openings in the leaves that connect to thin water tubes (xylem tubes) that run all the way down to the roots. The evaporation creates a vacuum at the top of the xylem tubes. How does the giant sequoia apparently violate the 33-foot limit described above?

Answers

19.1 The position of the pressure transducer doesn't matter because, in the absence of gravity, there is no hydrostatic pressure component. The column of fluid in the pressure measurement tubing exerts no force (it has no weight in space).

19.2 No. For venous air embolism to occur, subatmospheric pressure must exist within the perforated blood vessel. Subatmospheric pressure can be generated within a blood vessel in 2 ways. One, blood inside the vessel must be elevated above the heart; however, this generates subatmospheric pressure only in the presence of gravity. Two, the patient makes strong inspiratory efforts and the subatmospheric pressure in the thorax is transmitted into the blood vessels that drain into the chest. If the patient is mechanically ventilated (a likely scenario during brain surgery), the thoracic pressures will always be atmospheric or greater. Thus, a "vacuum effect" cannot be exerted on the blood vessels draining into the thorax.

Extra credit There is no theoretical height limit for a water column sustained by positive pressure from below (as opposed to suction from above). That's how well pumps work when the well is more than 33 feet deep. In the case of the giant sequoia, though, positive pressure is not generated from below. Instead, water is raised through capillary action because the xylem tubes are very narrow. Capillary action, nature's way of reducing surface tension, is not limited by atmospheric pressure.

INDEX

ABG measurements. *See*
arterial blood gas
measurements
adenosine diphosphate
(ADP), 89–90
adenosine triphosphate
(ATP), 89–90
ADP. *See* adenosine
diphosphate
afferent arm, in homeostasis,
143
afterload, in vascular
pressure, 45
air embolism, 23
causes, 33
alveolar air equation, 14–15
atmospheric pressure
and, 15
water vapor in, 15
alveolar compliance curve,
105, 107
influence of gravity on,
126
alveolar oxygen pressure
(P_{AO_2}), 14–15
estimation equation for,
14–15
hypoxemia and, 14
oxyhemoglobin dissociation
curve and, 15
alveolar pressure, 14–15
for oxygen, 14–15
alveolar ventilation, 101
arterial carbon dioxide
and, 102

anatomic dead space,
103–104
Fowler method for
determining, 103–104
anesthesiology, 95–96
aneurysm, 71
aortic arch baroreceptor, 4–5
Aristotle, 122, 123
arterial blood gas (ABG)
measurements, 109,
108–110, 120
for hypoxemia, 14–15, 111
oxyhemoglobin
dissociation curve
in, 110
arterial carbon dioxide, 101
alveolar ventilation and, 102
variables affecting, 107
arterial oxygen pressure
(Pa_{O_2}), 12
arterial-to-venous pathway, 41
atmospheric pressure, 13–14
alveolar air equation and, 15
ATP. *See* adenosine
triphosphate
atrial pressure, in giraffes, 30
autonomic nervous system,
pressure in, 5
avian pulmonary function.
See birds, pulmonary
circulation in

Badeer, Henry, 30–31
bar-headed goose, 129, 130
barometers, 8

development of, 6–7
mercury in, 7, 8
water, 9
Bernard, Claude, 141
Bernoulli, Daniel, 1
Bernoulli principle, 2–3
birds, pulmonary circulation
in, 129–132
bar-headed goose, 129, 130
countercurrent exchange
in, 130, 131, 134
crosscurrent exchange in,
131, 134
hyperventilation for, 129
ventilation/perfusion ratio
in, 130, 134
blood flow rates, circulatory
pressures and, 66
stressed volume, 72
unstressed volume,
71–72
blood pressure. *See also*
vascular pressure
cardiac output as influence
on, 78
during circulatory arrest,
70–71, 79
during circulatory arrest,
under Pascal's
principle, 70
decay curve, 80, 154
in giraffes, 36–37
mean arterial pressure, in
head, 41
Poiseuille's Law and, 37

blood pressure (continued)
  systemic circulation
    distance and, 80
    systolic, 72
blood volume
  during cardiac arrest, 84
  during circulatory
    arrest, 73
  pathologic vasodilation
    and, 72
  positional changes and, 72
  in zero-gravity, 153
Bohr, Christian, 103
Bohr equation, 102–104
  for dead-space volume,
    102, 103
bombardier beetle, 146
Burton, A.C., 3

Cannon, Walter, 142
capillary edema, 80–81
capillary overflow, 84. See
    also edema
carbon dioxide
  arterial, 101
  diffusion limitation for, 140
  PFTs for, 117
cardiac arrest
  acute tamponade and, 87
  blood pressure during,
    70–71, 79
  blood volume during, 84
  capillary edema and, 80–81
  capillary overflow and, 84
  cardiovascular system
    during, 82–85
  edema and, formation of,
    81–82
  hypothermia during, 70
  interventricular
    dependence after, 83–84
  mean systemic pressure
    during, 72
  pathologic vasodilation
    after, 72
  peripheral edema and, 81
  pressure and, 70–74
  pressure gradients
    during, 71

stressed blood volume
    during, 72
  unstressed volume during,
    71–72
  vessel pressure after, 81
cardiac output, 55. See also
    Starling's law of the
    heart
  blood pressure and, 78
  blood volume changes
    and, 58–59
  curve, 57
  inotropic increases and, 59
  left ventricular pressure
    in, 62
  venous return and,
    56–58
cardiovascular system.
    See also blood
    pressure; cardiac
    output; vascular
    pressure
  blood flow rates and, 66
  capillary overflow in, 84
  circulatory pressures
    and, 66
  during cardiac arrest,
    82–85
  frictional heat in, 11
  in giraffes, 27–31
  interventricular
    dependence in, 83–84
  perfusion pressure and, 26
  pressure in, 5
  total fluid energy in, 3–4
  venous return in, 48–52
carotid body chemoreceptor,
    144
  feedback loop, 144
carotid sinus baroreceptor,
    4–5, 144
causality, correlation and, 69
cellular metabolism, 89
  energy cascade for, 89
cerebral circulation, 32–33
  as closed circuit, 35
  in giraffes, 38
  hydrostatic pressure in, 35
  siphon effect in, 32–33, 38

transmural pressure in,
    35–36
  zones for, 35
cerebral perfusion pressure,
    35–36
  transmural pressure and,
    35–36, 152
chemiosmotic hypothesis,
    90, 93
chronic obstructive
    pulmonary disease
    (COPD), 108
circulatory arrest. See also
    cardiac arrest
  blood volume during, 73
  controlled, 73–74
  hypothermia and, 70, 73
  right atrial pressure
    during, 76
circulatory systems. See also
    cardiovascular system;
    venous return
  in giraffes, 27–31
  models, 34
  siphon systems in, 29–30,
    35
  in zero-gravity, 151–152
content pressure, 96
contractility. See inotropy, in
    venous return
controlled circulatory arrest,
    73–74
  arterial pressure with,
    77–78
  under Starling, 77
  vital signs during, 74
COPD. See chronic
    obstructive pulmonary
    disease
correlation, causality
    and, 69
countercurrent exchange,
    in birds, pulmonary
    circulation, 130,
    131, 134
crosscurrent exchange,
    in birds, pulmonary
    circulation, 131,
    131, 134

dead-space volume, 101, 103
  anatomic, 103–104
  Bohr equation for, 102, 103
  physiologic, 103
death, cell activity and, 88–89
diffusion limitation, 135–138
  for carbon dioxide, 140
  equilibrium in, 136–137
  Fick's law of diffusion and, 135–136
  membrane resistance in, 136, 140
  oxyhemoglobin dissociation curve and, 137–138
  perfusion limitation and, 140
  solubility of gases and, 138
diffusion-limited gases, 118

edema
  capillary, 80–81
  formation of, 81–82
  interstitial pressure and, 82
  oncotic pressure and, 82
  peripheral, 81
efferent arm, in homeostasis, 143
elastance, in vascular pressure, 43
energy
  for physiologic measurements, 11
  pressure and, 1, 11
  total fluid, 1, 2
Escher, M.C., 49, 50

FADH$_2$. *See* flavin adenine dinucleotide
feedback loop, in homeostasis, 144–146
  afferent arm in, 143
  carotid body chemoreceptor, 144
  components, 148

efferent arm in, 143
  positive, 148
Fick, Adolph, 94
Fick principle, 91, 95, 97, 99
  in anesthesiology, 95–96
  oxygen transport under, 96, 99
  oxyhemoglobin dissociation curve under, 96
Fick's law of diffusion, 91, 94–95, 97, 99
  blood oxygenating membrane size and, 99
  diffusion limitation, 135–136
  Ohm's law and, 94–95
  PFTs under, 118
flavin adenine dinucleotide (FADH$_2$), 89
flow rates
  in blood, circulatory pressures and, 66
  hydrostatic pressure and, 63
  for paddle wheels, 64
  pressure and, 63–67
  pressure gradients and, 69
  venous return influenced by, 65
flow-volume loop, 113, 112–117
  alveolar expansion and contraction, 115, 114–115
  for obstructive lung diseases, 113, 112, 116
  time constraints, 112–114
fluid density, hydrostatic pressure and, 19
Fowler method, 103, 104
frictional heat, 11

giraffes, 27–31
  atrial pressure in, 30
  cerebral circulation pressure in, 38
  circulatory physiology of, 27–31

high blood pressure in, 36–37
  jugular vein pressure components for, 31
  siphon systems in, 29–30
gravity, influence on lung ventilation, 104–105
  alveolar compliance curve, 105, 126
  in pulmonary circulation, 124, 125
Guyton, Arthur, 49, 55, 65, 74. *See also* venous return

Habeler, Peter, 12
hemodynamic properties
  invasive lines for, 5
  transducers for, 5
homeostasis, 142–146
  afferent arm in, 143
  in autonomic system, 144–145
  with carotid body chemoreceptor, 144
  efferent arm in, 143
  feedback loop, 144–146
  function of, 142
  in simple machines, 142–143
hydrostatic pressure, 19–24
  air embolism and, 23
  body of water and, size of, 21
  in cerebral circulation, 35
  development of, 63
  flow rates and, 63
  fluid density and, 19
  Pascal's principle for, 21, 26
  perfusion pressure, 22
  in siphons, 21–22
  transmural pressure, 22
  vertical distance and, 19
  in zero-gravity, 151
hyperventilation, in birds, 129
hypothermia, circulatory arrest and, 70, 73
  cell activity during, 88–89

hypoxemia, 14
    physiologic causes of,
        14–15, 111

inotropy, in venous return, 59
    left ventricle pressure
        and, 62
interstitial pressure, 82
invasive lines, 5
isovolemic contraction,
    44–45
isovolemic relaxation, 43

law of conservation of
    energy, 2–3. *See also*
        Bernoulli principle
left ventricular pressure, 62
Levy, Matthew, 65, 69
Lofting, Hugh, 56
lungs. *See* obstructive lung
    diseases; pulmonary
    circulation; ventilation,
    in lungs

MAP. *See* mean arterial
    pressure
mean arterial pressure (MAP)
    in head, 41
        system vascular resistance
            in, 48–49
        in venous return, 48,
            50–51
mean systemic pressure,
    50–51, 59
    during cardiac arrest, 72
measurements. *See also*
    barometers
    physiologic, energy
        necessary for, 11
    for pressure, 4–8
    Torr, 8
Messner, Reinhold, 12
Mitchell, Peter, 89, 90
    chemiosmotic hypothesis,
        90, 93
mitochondria, oxygen in,
    89–90
    through ATP, 89–90
muscle wasting, 151

NADH. *See* nicotinamide
    adenosine dinucleotide
nicotinamide adenine
    dinucleotide (NADH), 89

obstructive lung diseases,
    113, 112, 116. *See also*
    chronic obstructive
    pulmonary disease
    types of obstructions in,
        115–116
    variable intrathoracic, 117
Ohm's law, 51
    Fick's law of diffusion
        and, 94–95
oncotic pressure, 82
oxygen, 88–91
    cell diffusion of, 90–91
    in cellular metabolism, 89
    chemiosmotic hypothesis
        for, 90, 93
    diffusion limitation for,
        135–138
    in energy cascade, for
        cellular metabolism, 89
    under Fick principle,
        96, 99
    in mitochondria, 89–90
    oxidization characteristics
        of, 90–91
    schematic pathway for,
        91, 97
oxyhemoglobin dissociation
    curve, 15
    in ABG measurements, 110
    diffusion limitation and,
        137–138
    under Fick principle, 96

Pao$_2$. *See* arterial oxygen
    pressure
PAO$_2$. *See* alveolar oxygen
    pressure
partial pressure, 96
Pascal, Blaise, 7
Pascal's principle, 21, 26
    blood pressure under,
        during circulatory
        arrest, 70

Pasteur, Louis, 142
pathologic vasodilation, 72
PB. *See* pressure, barometric
perfusion limitation, 140
perfusion limited gases, 118
perfusion pressure, 22
    across arterial-to-venous
        pathway, 41
    blood flow and, 26
    cerebral, 35–36
    in siphons, 32
    transmural pressure
        and, 26
Périer, Florence, 7
peripheral edema, 81
PFTs. *See* pulmonary
    function tests
physiologic dead space, 103
*Physiology and Biophysics
    of the Circulation*
    (Burton), 3
Piper, Johannes, 131
pneumothorax, lung
    ventilation and,
    105, 107
Poiseuille's Law, 37
positive feedback loop, 148
preload, in vascular
    pressure, 44
pressure. *See also* mean
    arterial pressure
    alveolar, 14–15
    atmospheric, 13–14
    atrial, in giraffes, 30
    in autonomic nervous
        system, 5
    barometer, development
        of, 6–7
    barometric (PB), 12
    in cardiovascular system, 5
    circulatory arrest and,
        70–74
    content, 96
    definition of, 1
    energy and, 1, 11
    flow and, 63–67
    hydrostatic, 19–24
    in interstitium, 82
    mean systemic, 50–51

measurement of, 4–8
oncotic, edema formation
and, 82
partial, 96
perfusion, 22
right atrial, 48–49,
55–60
transducers and, for
measurement of, 5
transmural, 22
vascular, 42–45
pressure gradients
during circulatory
arrest, 71
flow rates and, 69
for paddle wheels, 64
for venous return, 54
pulmonary circulation,
122–126. *See also*
ventilation, in lungs
in birds, 129–132
function of, 122–123
influence of gravity on,
124, 125
as low-pressure system,
123–124
Starling resistor in, 125
ventilation/perfusion ratio
in, 128
in zero-gravity, 126
zones for, 125–126
pulmonary function tests
(PFTs), 108–118
ABG measurements, 109,
108–110, 120
for carbon dioxide
diffusion, 117
for COPD, 108
for diffusing capacity, 117
under Fick's law of
diffusion, 118
flow-volume loop, 113,
112–117
with spirometry, 111–112

respiratory quotient, 12
Ricci, Michelangelo, 7
right atrial pressure, 48–49,
55–60

blood flow rate and, 66
blood volume changes
and, 58–59
cardiac output and, 55
during circulatory
arrest, 76
inotropic increases
and, 59
under Starling's law,
55, 57
tamponade effects on, 79
volume loading in, 58

Scheid, Peter, 131
siphons
in cerebral circulation,
32–33, 38
with collapsible tubing
systems, 38
in giraffe circulatory
system, 29–30
as gravitationally
neutral, 35
hydrostatic pressure in,
21–22
limb diameter and, 23
perfusion pressure in, 32
transmural pressure in, 32,
33–34
Sonnenblick, E.H., 78
spirometry, 111–112
normal values for, 112
spirograms, 111
Starling, Ernest, 77
controlled circulatory
arrest and, 77
lectures, 78
Starling forces, edema
formation and, 81–82
Starling resistor, 125
Starling's law of the heart,
55, 57, 77–85
The Story of Doctor Dolittle
(Lofting), 56
stressed blood volume, 72
during trauma, 72
stroke volume, vascular
pressure and, 43
changes in, 45

left ventricle pressure
and, 62
system vascular resistance,
48–49
systolic pressure, 72

tamponade
cardiac arrest and, 87
circulatory pressure
influenced by, 79
time constraints, in flow-
volume loop, 112–114
definition, 114
Torr, as measurement of
mercury, 8
Torricelli, Evangelista, 6
barometer, development
of, 6–7
total fluid energy, 1, 2
in cardiovascular system,
3–4
transducers, 5
transmural pressure, 22
in cerebral circulation,
35–36
cerebral perfusion pressure
and, 35–36, 152
perfusion pressure and, 26
in siphons, 32, 33–34

unstressed volume, 71–72

vascular pressure, 42–45
afterload changes
in, 45
determinants of, 43
elastance in, 43
inotropic changes in, 44
isovolemic relaxation, 43
isovolumic contraction,
44–45
phases of, 42
preload changes in, 44
stroke volume in, 43, 45
volume loops in, 44
vascular waterfall. *See*
Starling resistor
venous return, 48–52
blood flow rate and, 66

cardiac output and, 56,
57–58
curve in, 51–52, 57
downstream pressure
in, 49
flow rate as influence
on, 65
inotropic increases in, 60
MAP in, 48, 50–51
mean systemic pressure
in, 50–51, 59
Ohm's law in, 51
pressure gradient for, 54
right atrial pressure,
48–49
system vascular resistance
in, 48–49
tamponade effects
on, 79
upstream pressure in, 49
ventilation, in lungs,
101–105. *See also*
pulmonary function
tests (PFTs)

alveolar, 101
alveolar compliance curve
for, 105, 107
arterial carbon dioxide
in, 101
Bohr equation, 102–104
dead-space volume and,
101, 103
gravity influence on,
104–105
physiology of, 102
in pneumothorax, 105, 107
ventilation/perfusion
ratio, 128
in bird pulmonary
circulation, 130, 134
vertical distance, hydrostatic
pressure and, 19
vital signs, during controlled
circulatory arrest, 74
Viviani, Vincenzo, 6

water barometers, 9
Waterfall (Escher), 50

water vapor, 15
partial pressure for, 18
as temperature
dependent, 18
West, John, 13

zero-gravity
blood pressure decay
curve with, 154
blood volume in, 153
cerebral perfusion
pressure in, 152
circulatory systems in,
151–152
hydration status in, 153
hydrostatic pressure
in, 151
muscle wasting with, 151
physiologic functions
with, 149–154
pulmonary circulation
in, 126
transmural pressure
in, 152